# Practicing Prodependence

In *Practicing Prodependence: The Clinical Alternative to Codependency Treatment*, Drs. Weiss and Buck present a new social and psychological model of human interdependence-focused treatment for families and loved ones of addicts.

Unlike Codependence, Prodependence celebrates the human need for and pursuit of intimate connection, viewing this as a positive force for change. This strength and attachment-based model is focused on accepting and celebrating human connection in ways that are healthy and life affirming for each person – even in the face of addiction. In this way, Prodependence presents a new paradigm through which loved ones can learn to love more effectively, without bearing shame or judgment for the valuable help they give.

This book will assist counselors, therapists, and addiction professionals in improving the ways they treat loved ones of addicts and other troubled people, teaching readers how to offer clients more dignity for their suffering than blame for the problem.

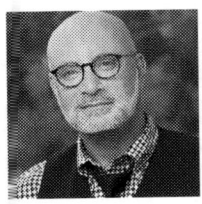

**Rob Weiss, PhD, LCSW**, is Chief Clinical Officer of Seeking Integrity LLC, working with sex, porn, and substance/sex-addicted men. He is an expert in the treatment of adult intimacy disorders and related addictions. A clinical sexologist and practicing psychotherapist, he has created intimacy-focused clinical treatment programs in the US, overseas, and for the US military. He serves as a subject matter expert for major media outlets including CNN, NPR, The New York Times, and Newsweek, among others. He is the author of ten books, including *Prodependence*, *Sex Addiction 101*, and *Out of the Doghouse*. His *Psychology Today* blog, "Love and Sex in the Digital Age," has had over 20 million readers, while his podcast, "Sex, Love, and Addiction," has generated more than 900,000 eager listeners since its inception in 2019.

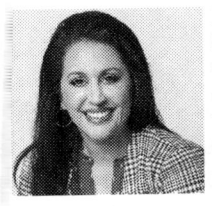

**Kim Buck, PhD, LPC**, is the owner of Aspire Counseling Services and an executive team member at Family Strategies Counseling Center. Dr. Buck is a practicing licensed professional counselor and clinical sexologist, who is highly specialized in the treatment of adult problematic sexual behaviors and the challenges associated with intimate betrayal. She creates curriculum, trains and supervises clinicians, and educates the public in a variety of forums. She gratefully serves as a clinical consultant to the HOPE Mental Health Foundation (501(c)(3)) that raises funds to provide specialized mental health services to local underserved communities. Kim resides in Arizona with her husband of 31 years, and together they have two adult children.

# Practicing Prodependence

The Clinical Alternative to Codependency Treatment

**Rob Weiss and Kim Buck**

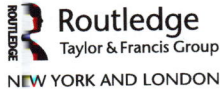
Routledge
Taylor & Francis Group

NEW YORK AND LONDON

First published 2022
by Routledge
605 Third Avenue, New York, NY 10158

and by Routledge
4 Park Square, Milton Park, Abingdon, Oxon, OX14 4RN

*Routledge is an imprint of the Taylor & Francis Group, an informa business*

*Library of Congress Cataloging-in-Publication Data*
Names: Weiss, Robert, 1961– author. | Buck, Kim, author.
Title: Practicing prodependence : the clinical alternative to
    codependency treatment / Robert Weiss, PhD, Kim Buck, PhD.
Description: New York, NY : Routledge, 2022. | Includes bibliographical
    references and index.
Identifiers: LCCN 2021048846 (print) | LCCN 2021048847 (ebook) |
    ISBN 9780367527822 (hardback) | ISBN 9780367527808 (paperback) |
    ISBN 9781003058359 (ebook)
Subjects: LCSH: Codependency.
Classification: LCC RC569.5.C63 W36 2022 (print) |
    LCC RC569.5.C63 (ebook) | DDC 615.5—dc23/eng/20211117
LC record available at https://lccn.loc.gov/2021048846
LC ebook record available at https://lccn.loc.gov/2021048847

ISBN: 978-0-367-52782-2 (hbk)
ISBN: 978-0-367-52780-8 (pbk)
ISBN: 978-1-003-05835-9 (ebk)

DOI: 10.4324/9781003058359

Typeset in Times New Roman
by Apex CoVantage, LLC

Access the Support Material: www.routledge.com/9780367527808

All illustrations are by Ashlynn Mya Jones except the drama triangle illustration.

To anyone who has ever felt responsible for someone else's addiction.

May this work set you free.

# Contents

# Foreword

Clinically oriented terms and ideas commonly get co-opted by popular culture ways that can promote unnecessary divisiveness and blame. Most social scientists pursue concepts and terminology that seek to better understand the human experience. It is also very human to use these ideas and terms to explain one's own suffering. Unfortunately, it is also very human to then point to other people as *the central cause* of one's own suffering. This can lead to blame, name-calling, and demonization. Our tendency as human beings to make meaning of our experience, combined with our need to protect our interests when under stress or in distress, can lead to feelings such as "I'm so unhappy, and I don't know why. Wait, I *do* know why. It's because of *you*." Sadly, these very human traits rooted in the evolutionary imperative to protect ourselves and our communities from external threats can also lead people to blame and adversity, rather than bonding and affiliation.

The term *Codependency* is one such example. What began in the 1980s as a harmless description of an interpersonal dynamic between an alcoholic who overfocuses on alcohol, and a partner who overfocuses on the alcoholic and the alcoholic's drinking, has devolved into a nasty, divisive rant in the public sector, one that tends to question rather than celebrate our natural need for meaningful dependency. When applied to psychotherapy and counseling in the 21st century, *Codependency* has become a misleading and destructive term that runs counter to our attachment-sourced research and beliefs about human relationships. It is time, as suggested throughout this text that the term Codependence be retired from our clinical lexicon and replaced by more compassionate and relationally balanced beliefs and language.

Our need to attach to at least one other human being is something of a biological imperative, one we cannot ignore. Our need to attach to others is linked to survival. For instance, an infant cannot survive without a postnatal umbilical to an older human caregiver. Humans therefore begin with dependency and that dependency on another human being or beings is a necessary condition for survival. We can argue that we are dependent on others from the beginning of life and dependent upon others toward the end as well. But what of the in-between? Are we fundamentally dependent creatures? We might say yes... and no. True helplessness requires a measure of dependency on others, and this is true at the beginning of life and at the end of life. Between the beginning and end of our lives, we learn to be independent, autonomous, and self-sufficient. We form unions with others ideally based on equality, shared purpose, shared meaning, and shared rules on how we will behave, particularly when under stress and distress. These adult unions function best when partners view themselves as *interdependent*.

In a union based on interdependence, people realize they are mutual stake-holders in all shared outcomes. In a free society of equals, partners unionize around shared interests in survival as well as thriving and prospering. There-fore, each partner has the same to lose and the same to gain and this provides them with equal power and authority over the other. Any other system would be dictatorship or slavery. We might call these systems *secure functioning* – meaning, partners are a team and are fully collaborative and cooperative with each other. They are driven by purpose and principle in their goals and attain-ment of absolute safety and security at all times – with mistakes, of course. In other words, they operate as a two-person system. One-person systems are too non-collaborative, too pro-self, too unfair, unjust, and insensitive too much of the time. These structures will always build resentment and threat because they represent insecure functioning.

Rigidly independent persons may *not* in fact be truly independent but are instead fearful or contemptuous of their own dependency needs as learned in their family of origin. These individuals are frightened of perceived threats to their freedom and autonomy. Similarly, overly dependent persons may be afraid of their own autonomy and their right to a fully equal, fair, and just partnership fearing enmeshed loss or abandonment. Interdependence is only possible if both individuals respect and acknowledge their basic dependency and autonomy needs. Truly interdependent partners neither fear, dismiss, nor devalue needs for independence or dependence in themselves or the other.

Arguments surrounding independence versus dependence are mostly false by popular definition. Interdependence is the result of two or more adults com-ing together as separate, autonomous individuals who *depend* on each other for reasons *other than feelings*. A shared purpose to protect each other from harm *is* a reason to interdepend. Our reasons to interdepend as autonomous individu-als rests upon our shared purpose, shared goals, and agreed-upon principles as to how we will govern each other. In other words, interdependent partnerships involve two or more people *of equal power and authority*, shared stakeholders who operate cooperatively, collaboratively, and in a manner that is fair, just, and sensitive to each other's differences and sensibilities – independent yet responsible to the union that protects and serves their interests.

In his book *Prodependence: Moving Beyond Codependency*, Rob Weiss properly argues that the term *Codependency* no longer holds its original mean-ing and intent. He further suggests this term has become so pejorative and ubiquitous as to be misleading, even damaging to those who use and iden-tify with its various meanings. Throughout this clinical follow-up, the authors expertly guide the reader to greater insight into interdependence, our natural,

healthy human need to depend on others in balance with our wish to simultaneously remain independent and autonomous known as *interdependency*.

As you read and use this insightful, practical work by Drs. Weiss and Buck,
rejoice in the human capacity to both depend and interdepend on other human
beings as relationships are unquestionably our most valuable commodity
throughout life and the one domain where we will always find meaning and
purpose.

*Stan Tatkin, PsyD, MFT – Co-founder of the PACT*
*Institute and author of* We Do: Saying Yes to a
Relationship of Depth, True Connection, and Enduring Love

# Preface

In 1909, Charles Darwin published his now-acknowledged masterwork, *The Origin of Species*, with an introduction stating that his book was, more than anything else, *his opinion*, based primarily on his experience and observations as a naturalist, geologist, and biologist.

> This Abstract, which I now publish, must necessarily be imperfect . . . and I must trust to the reader reposing some confidence in my accuracy. No doubt errors will have crept in, though I hope I have always been cautious in trusting to good authorities alone. I can here give only the general conclusions at which I have arrived, with a few facts in illustration, but which, I hope, in most cases will suffice. No one can feel more sensible than I do of the necessity of hereafter publishing in detail all the facts, with references, on which my conclusions have been grounded; and I hope in a future work to do this.[1]

He hoped that his theories would be received with an open mind and thus investigated by other scientists over time. Darwin well understood that his ideas were likely to be met with strong resistance and objections on many fronts. Despite the criticism and professional outrage he knew his writing might evoke, he unquestionably felt that such personal concerns were outweighed by the benefits his work could bring to science and to humanity as a whole. We suspect that if Darwin were alive today to witness the still ongoing creationism vs. evolution debate, he would not regret the publication of his work. In fact, we think he might say something like, "If we do not push forth and test new theories, we do not learn and grow."

With the publication of this book, we find ourselves in a similar circumstance – pushing forth an entirely new clinical belief system based on preliminary investigation and personal experience combined with extensive feedback offered us by many other seasoned addiction professionals. As Darwin did with *The Origin of Species*, the authors of this work have relied upon a considerable amount of existing data; however, this work is ultimately conceptual in nature, written to encourage clinicians to consider new ways of thinking and working, which may lead to more effective treatment outcomes. Moreover, this book reflects our shared desire to develop a more compassionate and effective mental health and addiction treatment while encouraging extensive new research to help grow this work.

The authors of this text fully acknowledge that the new approach we espouse – Prodependence – is not a criteria-based diagnosis, nor is it a time-tested methodology. More importantly, *we do not believe it should ever become a diagnosis*. That is not the intent of our theories. Prodependence – a concept evolved from attachment theory – can be viewed as a synonym for healthy interdependent relationships as applied to individuals and families who are deeply, emotionally connected to active or newly recovering addicts as opposed to the predominant model, Codependence. We strongly believe that Prodependence will prove its worth, with time and validated research, as a preferred methodology for working with this population.

That said, at this time Prodependence is a concept in need of practice, evaluation, and research. To that end, we have outlined in this volume what we believe to be the definition, parameters, and best methodology of Prodependence treatment. Our hope is that the approach we outline in this book can and will be tested by both practicing psychotherapists and scholarly researchers, and that, as this occurs, the concept either will or will not stand the test of time.

Despite our extensive criticism and challenges herein to past treatment modalities, it is not our intention to diminish the work previously developed and published by other authors and clinicians. We view our field as ever-changing and continually evolving; thus, we seek to build upon the past as a foundation toward the future.

In closing, we very sincerely hope that this work will motivate some of you to begin the research and clinical work required to determine whether these ideas, beliefs, and styles of clinical engagement are useful or not, in whole or in part.

The ideas are here; their proofs lie ahead.

– Rob Weiss PhD, LCSW
– Kim Buck, PhD, LPC

# Acknowledgments

## Dr. Weiss – Acknowledgments

### Personal

There are those who have shown me that loving attachments are possible. Some of the people remain in my life today and some not. But I remain attached to them forever. To me that defines *family*. But my marriage to Jon has shown me that empathy, respect, and contentment can actually live *in my own home*! And for that and so much more – I am forever grateful.

### To My Coauthor

From the bottom of my heart, I want to thank my coauthor Dr. Kim Buck. She was the first to embrace and then structure Prodependence into viable clinical programming. Dr. Buck then made this work the foundation of her doctoral dissertation. And that brought us together to write this work. We got through this evolution together; I have no doubt that there is more to come.

### Professional

Special thanks to my professional colleagues at Seeking Integrity, Tami Ver-Helst, Stuart Leviton, Karen Brownd, Scott Brassart, and Dr. David Fawcett who have banded together to develop more effective and compassionate forms of addiction treatment. Thanks to Dr. Stan Tatkin for his generous and empathic support and our book's amazing forward. Thanks to Grace McDonnell and Amanda Devine at Routledge, Taylor & Francis who have believed in and cheered for this project from day one. Thanks to Dr. Carol Clark and the educational team of the International Institute of Clinical Sexology (IICS). A shout-out to Christian Blonshine and Christine Belleris and my friends at HCI Books. Props to Keith Arnold, Cheryl Brown, Rose Westerman, Cheryl Cambay, Charlie Risien, and all those who have offered me their insights and their love.

# Dr Buck – Acknowledgments

My center of gravity is and has always been my family. From loving parents, siblings, and beyond – I will forever be grateful for the experiences that formed me. Thank you to my husband Fred, for your endless support in my pursuits and while letting me fly, always creating the safest place to land. I love you. To Skylar and Bailey, thank you for continually teaching me how to love and listen. I stand in awe of you and being your mom is by far my favorite adventure. I am so proud of you both. To Nick and Rachel, how lucky and blessed I feel to have you in my circle. To all of my countless friends and associates – thank you for giving my life so much color and meaning.

To my coauthor, colleague, and friend Dr. Rob Weiss. Thank you for your courage to create and formulate Prodependence. I will forever be grateful for your mentorship, guidance, and confidence in me. Thank you most of all for helping me put into words what was written on my heart.

Thank you to Routledge, Taylor & Francis for believing in this project and specifically to Amanda Devine and Grace McDonnell for your guidance and patience on the journey of making it a reality. To the team at Seeking Integrity – for continuing to grow Prodependence and its influence across the globe. To Dr. Stan Tatkin for your thoughtful forward and belief in this new paradigm. To Scott Brassart for your organizing and editing genius. To my colleagues and friends at Family Strategies Counseling Center – thank you for your trust and help with implementing the Prodependence perspective within our programming. You have played a key role in the ongoing development and understanding of this concept.

Finally, a big shout-out to the brave pioneers of Prodependence who, even through their own heartache and pain, are laboring to establish a community where like individuals can connect and heal. You are the heart of this work.

## Note

1. Darwin, C. (1909). *The origin of species*. Dent.

# Section 1

# Understanding Codependence

# 1 The "Diagnosis" of Codependency

## Understanding Diagnoses

As longtime licensed mental health and addiction specialists, we need not question the need for universally agreed-upon diagnostic criteria and related treatment methods that are supported by valid research. Lacking such succinct guides, we could not provide effective, relevant clinical care. Like them or not, diagnostic guides like the Diagnostic and Statistical Manual of Mental Disorders (DSM) and International Classification of Diseases (ICD) provide clinicians with the common language required to define, share, and clearly understand various mental health diagnoses. Such guides also help us understand how and when such diagnoses can be effectively applied – the same as any medical health procedure.

Moreover, mental health and addiction professionals must have shared accurate language toward understanding a client's mental status. Within this diagnostic structure are guidelines toward how to best evaluate clients as they present. Well-organized psychological, psychiatric, and addiction counseling should always begin with the search for a working diagnosis while understanding that such diagnoses are forever evolving in sync with our understanding of the client. Accurate diagnoses offer clinicians a shared language informing us how to best proceed with directive, useful treatment. To this end, the DSM and ICD provide commonly accepted criteria and terminology, which in turn provides clinicians with a shared foundation for accurate treatment planning, documentation, and clinical work.

As stated, addiction and mental health providers cannot be fully effective without a common language regarding the issues our clients present. For example, if a therapist is temporarily treating a person who is in Baltimore for a few months, to do their best therapy, that clinician needs to receive accurate information from the client's home therapist in, say, Mississippi. For these therapists to accurately communicate about the client's needs, there must be a shared understanding of terms like bipolar disorder, depression, OCD, and all the rest. As our therapeutic goal is the provision of accurate, useful care to our mentally ill, psychologically challenged, and addicted clients, we must share a universal understanding of these diagnoses, along with common names for problems we treat.

DOI: 10.4324/9781003058359-2

## Problems with Diagnoses

Despite all that is stated earlier, many therapists don't fully agree with the rhetoric surrounding some diagnoses. In one example, the criteria given us to assess for personality disorders (borderline, narcissistic, and the like), which are described as *lifelong and chronic* by the DSM, often appear to arise more often from early-life complex attachment trauma and related emotional survival than any fixed personality problem. As such, our addiction and mental health diagnoses often reveal only a fraction of the larger issues being treated. Thus, they can miss the mark.

In fact, manuals like the DSM and ICD are written to describe what we see in front of us (what we see in the here and now), with little if any focus on where, how, or why these problems might have evolved. For example, the DSM provides no reason why someone has ended up with depression, OCD, narcissism, or addiction because the sole function of that text is to offer succinct, universally recognizable diagnostic criteria and labels that we can apply to define the problems most commonly addressed in psychotherapy and counseling.

We are not fans of *labeling* people, as all humans are complex and unique individuals who can never truly fit into any single category. Still, despite our personal beliefs and occasional frustrations regarding diagnostic tools like the DSM and ICD, we have never questioned the need for them.

## Diagnoses Change Over Time

Can diagnoses change? Yes, absolutely. In fact, therapists are ethically required to consistently review our working diagnoses and related treatment plans, altering and changing them as our experience of the client grows over time. That said, some diagnoses tend to be fixed and unchanging (often those that require psychiatric medication). Such diagnoses are likely to follow someone throughout their life span. Examples of fixed mental health diagnoses include bipolar disorder, schizophrenia, depression, and ADHD, to name but a few.

At the same time, we realize that many psychological concerns will shift and even disappear altogether as our work progresses and evolves. Our clients grow (or they do not), they get better (or worse), so our labels for their presenting problems will change accordingly.

Interestingly, it's not just personal diagnoses that can change. Diagnoses themselves can evolve.

Without question, *evolve* is the right word, as nearly all of us have witnessed many deeply held mental health beliefs deservedly tossed into the dustbin of history as more accurate truths were proven valid. In one obvious example, homosexuality, transgenderism, and fetishes were viewed as primary mental health disorders in the United States for over a century. It was only as validated research and societal norms advanced that we were able to gain new insights and beliefs, thus vastly improving the ways we evaluate and support human sexual health.

The very fact that we are asked to universally shift from prior belief systems to new ones based on ever-changing views of mental health is frustrating to some and downright upsetting to others. Understandably so. After all, change is never easy. But when seen in the larger picture, this ongoing process of clinical reevaluation and evolution on all levels provides the kind of insight and clarity that allows mental health and addiction care to be even more useful, safe, and effective. Every person treated brings us new truths. The fact that such *new truths* can be examined and explored leads to the growth of psychotherapy and addiction treatment.

## New Treatments Abound

There are constantly changing dynamics in the worlds of psychotherapy and addiction beyond the irregular diagnostic revisions offered up in the DSM and ICD. Every few years or so, some new therapy technique or concept, useful or not, lands with a splash in the clinical world, offering new ways to think about and implement various therapies. These new ideas often lead eager acolytes, aflame with enthusiasm, to boldly declare that they have found the latest and most effective way to provide therapy, counseling, trauma work, addiction treatment, etc.

In the early stages of such clinical trends, it's not unusual for some professionals to incorporate these new ideas into their practices (whether proven valid or not) and then enthusiastically tell all their peers about this great new therapy thing. And, in truth, as long as we practice ethically (have the patient's best interests in mind, do no harm, etc.), we are free to adopt any form of therapy that we think might be useful – proven or not. Thus, mental health and addiction treatment professionals and programs will often embrace new treatment trends, especially when they reflect meaningful changes in our societal and cultural beliefs.

Understandably, informed caregivers are always on the lookout for more productive ways to help. Thus, when presented with a therapy process purported to be faster, less painful, and more productive (especially one with deep cultural resonance), who wouldn't want to be first to jump on that bandwagon? We have made this leap ourselves at various points – including with Prodependence, the subject matter of this book.

Over the past half-century, clinicians have had to consider many new and evolving concepts, including dialectical behavioral therapy (DBT), eye movement desensitization and reprocessing (EMDR), somatic therapy, mindfulness, rebirthing, equine therapy, narrative therapy, Buddhist recovery, and on and on and on. Many of these methodologies have proven to be effective and have found their place in professional practice. Many others, including a few that seemed incredibly exciting and potentially useful in the moment, did not live up to expectations and faded away from practical application. Those not meeting validated standards of clinical work were discarded. Primal scream and Bataka bats leap to mind. Meanwhile, some of the more outré-sounding techniques – EMDR, for example – seemed a bit (or a lot) odd when introduced but now are well-validated and extremely useful.

At one time or another, all sorts of theories and practices have been embraced as viable, usually with well-defined methods (proven or not) for use. But sadly, as popular as many such clinical concepts and practices were at the time, a lot of these ideas have failed and been discarded. Exciting, new, and popular at the time? Yes. Effective? No.

A brief analysis of the evolution of trauma therapy reinforces these notions. Starting in the late 1960s, abreaction (emotional venting) was viewed as a primary therapeutic method for the treatment of trauma. Thus, any therapy that got clients crying, screaming, yelling, or (safely) expressing physical anger seemed like the way to go. Many therapists fully believed that these methods were essential ways to help people express and work through trauma, although many clients left our offices (and programs) more debilitated than when they arrived.

In this way, the passage of time, combined with useful research and experience, has taught us that many of these once new and exciting techniques are at best ineffective and, at worst, may create more trauma than they heal.

Today, we understand that meaningful trauma work is not primarily defined by abreaction but by a nurturing clinical relationship, internal and external boundaries, somatic work, DBT, and the like. The process of working with trauma survivors is far more articulated today than in the past as we now closely track our clients in their moment-by-moment experiences, rather than beginning with preconceived notions of what might help them. Trauma therapies now balance our clients' need for reflective insight into their experience with therapies that encourage emotional containment and stability.

In part, many past therapy methods seemed so right, even unassailable, because they deeply mirrored strongly held cultural beliefs and trends of the time. In the 1960s through the 1990s, for example, pop psychology trends strongly mirrored the Eurocentric beliefs and goals of the "Me Generation," which were strongly focused on self-actualization – the implicit goals being self-awareness, individuation, and personal growth.

The Me Generation was generally thought of as self-involved and narcissistic, particularly as commented upon by writers Tom Wolfe.[1] Younger people of the era (baby boomers) were generally thought to ascribe *more importance to self-fulfillment than social responsibility*. This attitude carried over into almost every aspect of American culture, including the world of psychotherapy.

Codependence, like many of the other concepts and techniques previously mentioned, evolved more from popular culture than from recognized clinical experience or research. As such, Codependency is a prime example of a hugely popular new idea that entered the therapy space while lacking the validated research to back it up (*then or now*). As trendy, well-timed concepts like Codependency become culturally dominant, they can also become entrenched in clinical practice before we've had time to fully evaluate their worth. Fortunately, such techniques are usually relatively quickly and easily discarded. But others, such as Codependence, can resonate so strongly with popular culture that they take on a life of their own. In one small example, at the time of this writing one can find more than 400 pop-culture, self-help, and clinical books on Codependency. And yet, many decades since its inception, we lack valid proof of the concept as well as any universally understood diagnostic criteria by which we can determine whether someone is Codependent. Thus, the obvious question arises: Which of the 400+ books on the topic is required reading for those who wish to accurately learn how to treat it? Even more importantly, what version of these should we be teaching the next generation of treatment professionals?

## When Compelling Trends Enter Clinical Work

Culture always profoundly influences how we view our work – sometimes in useful ways, sometimes not. In one small example, the Victorian period of the 19th century viewed women as soft, vulnerable creatures who needed protection (by men). To this point, women who got angry or expressed any other strong and therefore *culturally inappropriate* emotions were referred to as *hysterical*. Fainting was considered a sign of being overly emotional, even though corsets of the era left women little room to breathe, much less express strong emotions. No wonder they sometimes passed out. These misguided beliefs had far more to do with the rigid gender roles and views of sexuality of that period than with any validated facts.

In the psychotherapy world, it is only when cultural/clinical trends are validated by research-based facts that the rubber hits the road. Again, we will use the example of EMDR. When we first heard about EMDR, we were skeptical. How could eye movement lead to a reduction in trauma reactivity? But over time the science outweighed our skepticism; the facts became clear *in the research*. These days, EMDR is a proven, effective, and clinically validated form of trauma treatment. People who struggle with PTSD and other complex trauma issues have long needed a fast and effective way to reduce the intensity of their symptoms, and EMDR has delivered just that. In fewer than 15 years, EMDR went from a pop psychology trend to a deeply valued treatment modality.

This is the path we would expect of any theory that becomes universally integrated into the counseling world. Such concepts may start out as a trend, but with careful research and examination, they can become useful realities – but only as they are proven to be effective.

Science matters. Despite the comfort and familiarity many engaging concepts may offer us, such beliefs cannot rise to the level of a clinical diagnosis and a useful therapy method until proven to be true by scientific research. Without this process, every exciting new psychological concept, if perceived as truth, would send us spinning in a new direction – just because it felt right. And while good therapy does often stem from what feels right with a client, our diagnoses and related treatment plans cannot be determined by what feels right in the moment. Legitimate diagnoses and related treatment methods are created and confirmed by the best *facts* and information proved to be true over time.

Once again, we find ourselves bumping up against the concept of Code-pendency. Codependence is unquestionably one of those approaches that spread like wildfire, becoming entrenched in clinical thinking and practice and even spawning a 12-step program *without ever becoming a formally organized criteria-based diagnosis.*

## What Is Codependency?

Codependence, as commonly understood, occurs when one person tries to control the actions of another (in the guise of helping) so they can feel better about themselves and their relationship with that other person. The Codepend-ence model is rooted in discussions of early-life trauma and the ways in which such trauma can influence later life behaviors and relationships. Unfortunately, for many loved ones of addicts (and plenty of therapists), framing a person's commitment to helping a troubled loved one as stemming from that person's reignited early-life trauma (as opposed to being an expression of love and com-mitment) feels negative. Understandably, it feels to them as if they are being blamed, shamed, and pejoratively labeled for loving too much, or not in the right way, or for unconscious, selfish reasons.

This was likely not the original intent of the Codependence movement, but it's what we've currently got. The movement's progenitors were almost certainly not trying to say that loved ones of addicts provide loving care based solely on their own personal insecurities and neuroses (trauma repeti-tion). The originators of Codependence did, however, notice that most of the people in meaningful relationships with an addict did themselves have cha-otic and traumatic pasts. Unfortunately this observation was carried forward as a primary tenet of the Codependence model, which, in turn, led to many people feeling being blamed, shamed, and wrongly pathologized.

## How We Got Here

By the late 1980s, primarily with the release of six books, the term Code-pendence and the ideas surrounding it entered and became entrenched in the layperson's lexicon.

- In 1981, Claudia Black wrote *It Will Never Happen to Me: Children of Alcoholics as Youngsters–Adolescents–Adults.*[2]
- In 1982, Janet Woititz wrote *Adult Children of Alcoholics.*[3]
- In 1985, Robin Norwood wrote *Women Who Love Too Much: When You Keep Wishing and Hoping He'll Change.*[4]
- In 1986, Timmen Cermak wrote *Diagnosing and Treating Co-dependence.*[5]
- In 1986, Melody Beattie wrote *Codependent No More: How to Stop Con-trolling Others and Start Caring for Yourself.*[6]
- In 1989, Pia Mellody wrote *Facing Codependence: What It Is, Where It Comes From, How It Sabotages Our Lives.*[7]

In *Codependent No More*, Beattie identifies and addresses the pseudo-pathology that has long been attached to the Codependence model, writing, "Perhaps one reason some professionals call codependency a disease is because many codependents are reacting to an illness such as alcoholism."[8]

There is much impact in this statement. First, it indicates (in our opinion) that Beattie never intended for Codependency to be a pathology, that she was instead focused on gaining insight into the partner's experience. Next, it shows she realized, right from the start, that a lot of people would nonetheless view Codependence as pathology. So, even before Codependence became *a thing* in the collective mindset, Beattie sensed it would become pathologized.

Nowadays, the advice typically given by Codependence-oriented writers and therapists is that it's better for loved ones of addicts to detach and focus on caring for themselves – in particular, working to heal their own assumed trauma (the trauma that is said to underlie and drive their unhealthy caretaking) – than to focus on their troubled loved one. Or, as Beattie writes in *Codependent No More*, "Detach. Detach in love, detach in anger, but strive for detachment. I know it's difficult, but it will become easier with practice.... The focus is on you."[9]

## Why Codependence Struck a Chord

As stated earlier, the Codependence movement, once introduced, took off like a rocket. One reason for this was that it was the first readily accessible theory addressing the impact of addiction on the family. It identified addiction-driven family dysfunction as the powerful and profoundly impactful trauma that it is, and a whole lot of people identified with that. With Codependence, family members of addicts could finally view themselves, their feelings, and their behaviors through a lens that recognized and acknowledged the emotional effects of their loved one's addiction.

More importantly, like the self-actualization and women's rights movements that preceded and accompanied it, Codependence encouraged people (especially women) to empower themselves by focusing on themselves and their needs first, while setting better boundaries with others (especially the men in their lives). Women at the time were encouraged to eschew dependency on men, on love, on relationships, and on family, and to do less caregiving – focusing instead on their own needs and self-development. Unfortunately, the very beliefs that allowed women to push past many a glass ceiling spoke more to anti-dependence than independence or interdependence.

Inherent to Codependence is a simple message to women in relationships with challenging, demanding men (in this case, addicted men) – a message that tells them to detach from their troubled partner so they can focus on their own needs.

This new approach to relating gave women permission to differentiate as individuals – to take control of their own lives while simultaneously releasing control over their addicted loved ones (men). To a 1980s nation of women eager for equality, this message was readily received. The idea was both empowering and easily embraced.

## How Codependence Went Awry

Right from the start, Codependence was conflated with a long-established psychological disorder, dependent personality disorder. DPD is characterized by "a pervasive and excessive need to be taken care of that leads to submissive and clinging behavior and fears of separation, beginning by early adulthood and present in a variety of contexts."[10] For a DPD diagnosis, individuals must display five or more of the following criteria:

- Difficulty making everyday decisions without an excessive amount of advice and reassurance.
- Needing others to assume responsibility for most major areas of life.
- Difficulty expressing disagreement (based on fear of rejection and loss of support).
- Difficulty initiating projects or doing things on one's own.
- Going to excessive lengths to obtain nurturance and support from others, to the point of volunteering to do things that are unpleasant.
- Feeling uncomfortable or helpless when alone.
- Urgently seeking a new relationship as a source of care and support when one relationship ends.
- An unrealistic preoccupation with the fear of being left alone to take care of oneself.[11]

The simple truth is that the concept of Codependence quickly morphed – in the minds of the public, along with a large segment of the therapeutic community – into an unofficial pathology (that sounds a lot like DPD). This viewpoint is now so pervasive that if you go to the Wikipedia page for dependent personality disorder and scroll to the "See Also" section, the first hyperlink is to Wikipedia's page on Codependency – tangible evidence of how closely aligned the two terms have become in the public mind.[12]

Beattie, perhaps inadvertently, feeds this belief in *Codependent No More* by writing:

> When a codependent discontinued his or her relationship with a troubled person, the codependent frequently sought another troubled person and repeated the codependent behaviors with that new person. These behaviors, or coping mechanisms, seemed to prevail throughout the codependent's life – if that person didn't change these behaviors.[13]

Intentionally or otherwise, Codependency applies a pathological sheen to those who love and care for addicts and other deeply troubled, needful individuals.

It's like the world woke up one day and decided that displays of inherently powerful and traditionally feminine strengths like compassion, empathy, and caregiving were less important than the traditional male strengths of competitiveness, self-focus, and aggression. And based on that, both genders were taught, through the language of Codependence, that if you let someone else's needs meaningfully guide your actions, you are weak, they are dominant, and you will never become the best version of yourself.

That is not Codependence. That is anti-dependence.

According to Marion Solomon, espousing this perspective has only served to increase feelings of detachment and displeasure.

> The unfortunate solution that psychology books and psychotherapists offer to combat loneliness and isolation is to be strong enough to stand alone. In essence, we are exhorted: "Don't depend on others to love and affirm you. Know what you want. Find it within yourself. Be your own best friend. Heal yourself. Only then will you be mature and ready for love."[14]

Again, this was likely not the intention of the Codependency movement's progenitors. Nevertheless, caring for a troubled (especially an addicted) loved one has been slowly but steadily pathologized – if not officially, then in the collective mindset. In time, Codependence has come to mean caring for yourself *instead of* your addicted loved one, rather than caring for yourself *as well as* your addicted loved one.

Nowadays, people labeled as Codependent are often treated as if they have dependent personality disorder, even when their behavior does not even remotely approach that level of pathological neediness and enmeshment. Ross Rosenberg, author of *The Human Magnet Syndrome*,[15] discusses this unfortunate transition in a Psych Central article:

> Like other misunderstood and misused psychological expressions, "codependency" has taken on a life of its own. Once it went mainstream, it was haphazardly and conveniently reshaped to fit our mainstream vocabulary. Since its introduction in the 1980s, its meaning has devolved to describe a weak, needy, clingy, and even emotionally sick person.[16]

Rosenberg's statement may seem harsh, but it's absolutely on target. Codependence has evolved into a belief system that says caring for and trying to help another person, especially if that person is addicted, is, in and of itself, unhealthy, dysfunctional, and quite possibly pathological. Consider the following statement by counselor Scott Egleston, as quoted in *Codependent No More*: "Codependents are caretakers – rescuers. They rescue, then they persecute, then they end up victimized."[17] So, by definition, if/when we care for an addicted loved one, we place ourselves into one of the three positions on the famed Karpman Drama Triangle.

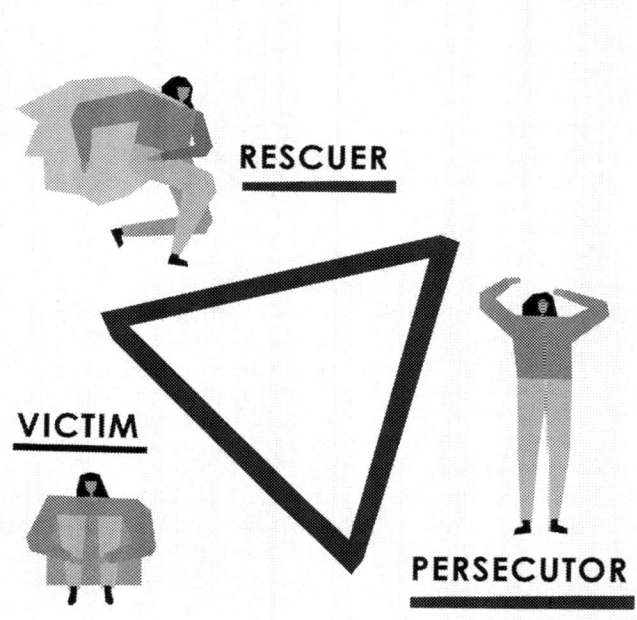

RESCUER

VICTIM

PERSECUTOR

To this end, spouses, parents, siblings, and friends of addicts are routinely counseled to focus on their own trauma-based weaknesses, to step away from their dysfunctional relationship with the addict, to stop rescuing, to stop ena-bling, to detach with love, and to just plain "stop being so codependent!"

Unfortunately, this approach does not empathetically meet such clients *where they are*. People with troubled loved ones are feeling anxious, fearful, out of control, and angry. Because of that, they often respond negatively to the themes of Codependency, as those themes innately feel wrong. Such individu-als will often respond with statements like, "How can I possibly abandon a person I love, especially in their hour of deepest need?"

And therein lies the problem. Codependency as a model does not meet loved ones of addicts where they are. Instead, it prejudges and labels them based on their understandable desires and attempts to help, and then, based on that prejudgment, it tells them what they are doing wrong and how to "fix it." As a result, many confused, overwhelmed, needful loved ones of addicts take away messages like:

- I am an active part of the problem.
- My attempts to care for my addicted loved one have made things worse.
- I am broken and defective and unworthy of a healthier relationship.
- I should have seen this coming.
- I don't know how to love someone.
- I shouldn't let myself be so affected by this. What's wrong with me?

Still, family members, friends, pastors, and well-educated therapists will work to convince a person who actively loves and cares for an addict that their willingness to put aside their own active lives to help a close other, someone they have likely loved (perhaps their entire life), is irrational, counterproductive, and a sign of *their own dysfunction*. Usually, these well-meaning advisors suggest therapy, interventions, and participation in support groups like CoDA as a way to more fully detach from a bad situation. Codependency has endless ways of informing such people that their desire to intervene on their loved one's problems is interfering with a necessary refocus toward their own needs, wants, and self-fulfillment.

## What Are Codependency Assessments Based Upon?

If you Google Codependence or read any of the 400+ books on the topic, you'll find endless lists delineating the core traits of Codependent people, several psychological assessments for Codependence, and a variety of self-tests for identifying the problem of Codependency. What you will not find is an official diagnosis for Codependency because that diagnosis does not exist. For decades, clinicians have been treating clients, especially loved ones of addicts, as if there were an official diagnosis for Codependence, but the research has never shown that Codependency treatment (however it is envisioned by its countless practitioners) has an overall positive impact on the caregiver, the addict, or the family.

The resources you do find when you research Codependency range from the ACoA's Laundry Lists to CoDA's Patterns and Characteristics of Codependence to Charles Whitfield's 38-item Likert-style checklist to the Spann-Fischer Codependency Scale to countless quizzes, lists, and tests provided in blogs, articles, and books on Codependence. The simple truth is that there is a lot of writing about Codependence but *no official diagnosis*. Instead, there is an unofficial pseudo-diagnosis linked, regardless of the source, to the following basic criteria:

- A Codependent person makes extreme sacrifices to satisfy the needs of a loved one.
- A Codependent person finds it difficult to say no when a loved one makes demands on their time and energy.
- A Codependent person covers or tries to manage a loved one's problems with alcohol, drugs, money, the law, etc.
- A Codependent person sublimates their needs to meet the needs of loved ones.

- A Codependent person is overly focused (to the point of obsession) on the well-being of their troubled loved ones.
- A Codependent person has poor boundaries about helping, often doing for addicts (and others) things those people should be doing for themselves.

People who behave in these ways tend to be "diagnosed" as Codependent. To us, however, these traits sound less like a pathology and more like a person who cares deeply about the well-being of a troubled loved one.

Ask yourself:

- Who doesn't make sacrifices for a person they love, especially if that person is struggling?
- Who doesn't say yes to a family member asking for assistance?
- Who doesn't try to help the family save face in difficult circumstances?
- Who wouldn't sublimate their needs to help a struggling loved one?
- Who doesn't worry obsessively when a loved one is struggling?
- Who hasn't overstepped healthy boundaries at least occasionally in an eager attempt to help a loved one?

To us, this is the primary failure of the Codependency model. As an analytic theory, it is more focused on the shortcomings of the caregivers and their unresolved, unconscious early-life traumas, rather than simply acknowledging their inherent strengths. We believe that working with this population requires more focus on providing validation, support, and direction in the *here and now* than on delving into the past. We believe that caregiving loved ones are simply doing the best they know how to love and rescue their broken families. To our thinking, any implication that such loved ones are somehow enabling or reinforcing the addictive process is both abusive and disrespectful to their efforts to maintain love and connection. Such caregivers are not causing or enabling the crisis; their efforts (right or wrong) are simply in the service of helping the loved one and family survive.

### The Survival of Love

Loving too much is not a disease. Providing support and nurturance is not unhealthy, nor is needing support and guidance. These are among the most important concerns of intimate, caring relationships. The perception that normal caretaking is inherently unhealthy must be reversed in our modern culture if love is to survive.[18]

### Addicts Require Addiction Treatment

Treatment for those who struggle with addiction has significantly advanced over the last 35 to 40 years, with a wide variety of models having evolved, the most effective of which are grounded in cognitive-behavioral theory.

In whatever way addicts are initially engaged in treatment, they nearly always need, first and foremost, a giant dose of reality. Once we have ensured that they are psychologically stable and appropriate candidates for addiction work, breaking through the façade of denial that allows them to engage in active addiction with little internal impunity is task number one. Little movement toward long-term change can occur until these clients understand and view their addiction as the destructive force that it is. In more formal terms, our job is to help shift the addicts' psychological relationship to their addiction from ego-syntonic (something they like and eagerly seek out) to ego-dystonic (something they dislike and wish to avoid).

Once denial unravels, which can be a difficult and time-consuming process, a plan for ongoing sobriety with a strong focus on honesty, trust-building, and accountability can be implemented. Usually, this plan incorporates a mix of individual therapy, addiction-focused group therapy, cognitive-behavioral work, social learning, and 12-step or similar support groups.

Many addiction professionals recognize that the disease of addiction is in great part a reflection of early attachment trauma. This belief implies that early injuries cause these wounded people to seek emotional regulation via addictive substances and behaviors, rather than leaning into healthy dependent relationships. This is why approaches that are inclusive of group therapy, 12-step recovery, and other support groups are often effective; they help lead addicts away from the isolation that defines addiction and toward supportive individuals and groups.

At some point, addicts are also asked to identify and eventually to address the underlying emotional deficits and trauma that lead them into addiction in the first place. At a minimum, reviewing a client's trauma history helps to reduce shame. Essentially, this work tells addicts,

> You're not an addict because you're a bad person. You're an addict because some bad things happened when you were younger, and you cleverly learned to escape your painful emotions by numbing out. Unfortunately, you're still handling your problems by escaping from them instead of turning to others for help. You are not bad, you are broken. And broken people can be fixed.

In this way, trauma is addressed throughout early therapy but not worked through until the client is stable (sober). In the early days of addiction recovery, the goal of helping these clients gain insight into their problematic past is used to help normalize the reasons why they have an addiction, thereby reducing shame and self-hatred.

Whichever approaches are embraced by the clinician providing treatment, the therapeutic work required for early addiction care looks something like this:

- Gain insight into client stability, history, and functioning.
- Engage in immediate and ongoing crisis management.
- Gain client trust via empathy, support, insight, and healthy goal setting.
- Strongly confront denial and the disordered thinking that feed the addictive process.

- Identify the addictive patterns, substances, and behaviors.
- Identify addiction triggers (the people, places, and things that precipitate a need/desire to use).
- Identify and provide alternatives to active addiction (healthier ways to cope with triggers).
- Examine past trauma – abuse, neglect, and other issues that have created an inability to trust and securely attach.
- Help reduce client shame by building an intellectual (if not emotional) relationship between their problematic early life history and their current addictive behavior.
- Encourage and validate earned security through interdependent connections with clinicians, fellow recovering addicts, friends, and, most importantly, loved ones.
- Repeat.

At the end of the day, treating addicts ultimately focuses on moving the client out of the denial that supports isolation and toward the development of healthy dependent relationships. Thus, a primary goal of all addiction treatment is to encourage and facilitate a transition from addictive dependency to effective interpersonal dependency.

## Effective Treatment Mirrors Client Need

Choosing the most useful treatment modality in any given case asks clinicians to combine their clinical knowledge and experience with continuously evolving assessments of the clients themselves. Armed with this information, we then choose the most effective approach for a specific client's presenting concerns. Our therapy modalities are never random. The form of care chosen is based on our education, experience, and accurate research in concert with clarity and insight into the presenting problem.

In one important example, the most effective form of treatment for people with behavioral problems (addiction is a good example) is founded in cognitive-behavioral work. Informed clinicians are not advised to address active behavioral problems (like addiction) with narrative, Jungian, analytic, somatic, or related self-reflective treatment modalities because such methods have proven ineffective. Treating active addicts requires us to organize treatment around cognitive-behavioral methods, putting aside psychodynamic and related work until clients are stable in their sobriety.

Well-trained clinicians don't just go with their gut, offer the types of treatment they are most comfortable providing, or shoehorn clients into preexisting treatment models that lack validity. Instead, they are careful to accurately match their methods to the presenting problem, the client's experience of that problem, the client's history and background, and informed counseling techniques. Should any case require a skillset that the clinician does not hold, they can learn how to adapt their work to meet the client's specific needs, or they can refer the client to someone more qualified to meet the client's needs.

## Are Caregivers Addicted Too?

Nearly all the current books and methodologies of Codependence, especially as applied to loved ones of addicts, have been created by individuals focused on the ways in which childhood trauma can (and often does) affect adult relationships and life. The general thinking is that people who end up loving, partnering with, and staying with addicts have experienced similar trauma in childhood, usually by growing up with an alcoholic, addicted, or mentally ill parent or caregiver. In this way, their involvement, care, and love for a troubled addict are seen as a form of trauma-repetition.

The basic tenet of Codependency is a belief that those who survive early-life dysfunction tend to carry that forward into their adult lives by bonding with and becoming dependent upon (even addicted to) troubled others who will, over time, neglect, abuse, and let them down in the same ways as their early caregivers. Clinically, these adult caregivers are then viewed as broken trauma survivors who are dragging past baggage into their current relationships.

This is one of the ways that Codependency fails such people, as it asks them to view themselves as *part of the problem* rather than part of the solution and then that becomes the focus of their care. The model tends to devalue and dismiss their current circumstances (an interpersonal crisis) by asking them what is wrong *with them* for being so reactive, over-engaged, and enmeshed. To make matters worse, Codependency encourages caregivers and other loved ones of addicts to view *themselves* as addicts too. In this way, their justifiably desperate attempts to fix and rescue an addicted loved one are viewed as a sign of their own addictive, trauma-derived pathology.

At this point, we ask you to consider:

- Can anyone really be addicted to a person?
- Can anyone truly love too much?
- Can the interpersonal dynamics (useful or not) in such relationships be judged or labeled when these caregivers are in the midst of a profound life crisis?
- Why judge or give a pathological-sounding label to those who are simply doing the best they can to keep their life together?
- Why consider them as anything other than caring, compassionate people whose pain, fears, and related behaviors are driven by the potential failure and loss of a deeply meaningful attachment?

Such views are mismatched to the experience of these people often causing them to feel like they are responsible for the addict's success or failure to achieve and maintain sobriety.

### No One Can Make an Addict Use

We cannot proceed without highlighting the fact that no one can make another person drink, use, or act out behaviorally. Ever. Burying oneself in addiction or returning to an addiction is a choice made by the addict. Loved ones of addicts may upset an addict, let an addict down, or even hurt an addict, but the way an addict chooses to cope is up to the addict.

Addicts always have choices. Whether they choose to return to alcohol, drugs, video gaming, porn, etc., or to reach out to empathic others for support is fully in their hands. No matter the hurt or anger of others, no matter how those feelings are expressed, no one other than the addict can ever carry the responsibility for active addiction.

## Codependency Shames the Victim

Viewing and telling the caregivers and other loved ones of broken people that they are obsessed with the pain, loss, trauma, and fear of losing their beloved other (as Codependency states) does not serve their more immediate needs for comfort, support, direction, and hope. Codependency simply does not meet such people *where they are* without prejudgment. To caregivers of addicts, the intellectual concept of Codependence simply doesn't feel native to their experiences. And why would it?

*Caregivers are not addicted to the ones they love!* Rather, they are loving people who are understandably obsessed with finding ways to return their loved one to health and family life. When we tell them that they are making the situation worse because they are acting out their own past trauma, thereby reinforcing the addiction, or we imply that they are addicted to the one they love, they feel blamed, shamed, misunderstood, and alienated. Sadly, this is not a path that leads these troubled people to feel as if they are compassionately and empathically understood by us. This is a problem.

If we view caregivers of active addicts as reenacting their own trauma by being addicted to their own troubled loved one, then we would logically provide them with therapy that mirrors the work we do with an addict. So, the focus of their care would then be to confront *their* denial, identify *their* problematic addictive patterns, all the while working to detach from the troubled person they love (i.e., to detach from their addiction). If they object to this way of thinking, Codependency tells them that this is yet another sign of their denial and, if this denial is not immediately addressed, they are likely to continue enabling the addict and the addiction. This too is a problem.

*We all have trauma issues* big and small that affect our adult behavior and relationship choices. But to focus on such insight-oriented work when the client in front of us is suffering here and now does not meet their needs and is out of sync with legitimate therapeutic training. Do these people have past issues worth exploration? Sure, we all do. Is it useful to point out those past problems when they are in a current crisis? Not at all.

## Loving Troubled People Is a Gift

No one gets a free ride. Drugs or no drugs, acting out or no acting out, we all experience trauma and loss from womb to tomb. The earlier the trauma and more enduring the wounds, the more problems we will face as adults, most profoundly reflected in our intimate relationships. This is a fact.

Our clients, especially spouses and family of addicts, are angered by this; they tell us, "But this is the opposite of everything you said. You told me that my past is not driving and supporting the addict's behaviors. You told me that I'm not part of the problem but part of the solution. I thought there was no Codependence." And there isn't.

Prodependence is about helping loved ones of addicts to move past *the early crisis stage* of another's addiction by making that the focus of treatment from day one. The authors do not intend to imply that loved ones don't have their own problems that might attract them to people with similar issues. We all do. Prodependence says, "Treat these people with dignity by not inviting them to enter insight-oriented psychotherapy or to view their love and care as an addiction when they are struggling to just get through the day!" Prodependence discourages clinicians from "going there" because there are more important and immediate issues on the table. Plus we need to remind ourselves that many clients have no interest in ever taking a deep dive into their early trauma, they just want things to get better. Prodependence further says that any client's decision to work on past concerns *after their lives have stabilized* is a personal choice – not a therapist's choice.

Many clients who are fed up with the Codependency model resent any implication that they are likely to bond with people who have similar early challenges to their own. What they don't understand is choosing who we love in part based on our past is a good thing and not a pathology! Building an intimate relationship with someone who has shared or mirrored issues to our own offers both of us the chance to grow and heal together.

Again Dr. Solomon:

> *We learn patterns of relating in early childhood and then tend to re-create them repeatedly in our lives. Indeed most partners choose each other with the unconscious hope of repeating what was good and repairing what was bad or lacking in their earliest relationships ... but early injury does not have to cause unhappy adult relationships. In fact nurturing our intimate*

> relationships in the present is the means by which emotional wounds from childhood can be healed.[19]

The following is how one of our clients reflected on this issue:

> What if I love him because I've seen the potential for us to grow together? What if I love and stay with him because I can see the better, more loving person he has been or might become. What if I hold out a vision of him at his best when everyone else sees only the bad. What if I am putting my life on hold to help solely because I love him? After all, I said *for better or for worse* How could that be wrong?

Codependency requires caregiving loved ones to gain insight into their own past trauma, and then these very facts are used against them as proof of how and why *they are addicted* to their troubled loved one. In essence, caregivers and other loved ones of addicts are told that there is *something wrong with them* based on who they have chosen to love and the ways they have chosen to deal with that person's illness. This allows no room to consider that they may have chosen the perfect person for them, regardless of their current circumstances.

Codependency treatment unfortunately asks counselors to see these people in the same light as the addict, leading to the logical conclusion that caregivers and other loved ones of addicts require the same kinds of therapies as addicts. This belief system can be viewed as unfair, even unethical (as there is no proof that such beliefs are actually true), which means that we have likely been missing out on effective care, with fewer meaningful, successful outcomes. Sadly, we have seen many such loving family members simply walk away from the help they desperately need because their Codependency-focused therapists have left them feeling more frustrated, angry, or ashamed than when they arrived.

## Notes

1. Wolfe, T. (1976). The me decade and the third great awakening. *New York Magazine, 23*(8), 26–40.
2. Black, C. (1981). *It will never happen to me: Children of alcoholics as youngsters–adolescents–adults*. Ballantine Books.
3. Woititz, J. G. (1990). *Adult children of alcoholics: Expanded edition*. Health Communications, Inc.
4. Norwood, R. (1986). *Women who love too much: When you keep wishing and hoping he'll change*. Simon & Schuster.
5. Cermak, T. L. (1986). *Diagnosing and treating co-dependence: A guide for professionals who work with chemical dependents, their spouses and children*. Johnson Institute Books.
6. Beattie, M. (1986). *Codependent no more: How to stop controlling others and start caring for yourself*. Hazelden Publishing.
7. Mellody, P., Miller, A. W., & Miller, J. K. (1989). *Facing Codependence: What it is, where it comes from, how it sabotages our lives*. Harper Collins.

8. Beattie, M. (1986). *Codependent no more: How to stop controlling others and start caring for yourself.* Hazelden Publishing.
9. Beattie, M. (1992). *Codependent no more: How to stop controlling others and start caring for yourself.* Hazelden Publishing.
10 American Psychiatric Association. (2013). *Diagnostic and statistical manual of mental disorders* (DSM-5®). American Psychiatric Publishing.
11 American Psychiatric Association. (2013). *Diagnostic and statistical manual of mental disorders* (DSM-5®). American Psychiatric Publishing.
12 Wikipedia. Dependent Personality Disorder. Retrieved March 8, 2018, from https://en.wikipedia.org/wiki/Dependent_personality_disorder
13. Beattie, M. (1992). *Codependent no more: How to stop controlling others and start caring for yourself.* Hazelden Publishing.
14. Solomon, M. (1994). *Lean on me: The power of positive dependency in intimate relationships.* Simon and Schuster.
15. Rosenberg, R. A. (2018). *The human magnet syndrome: The codependent narcissist trap.* CreateSpace Independent Publishing.
16. Rosenberg, R. A. (2013). *The history of the term codependency.* https://blogs.psychcentral.com/human-magnets/2013/11/the-history-of-the-term-codependency/
17. Beattie, M. (1992). *Codependent no more: How to stop controlling others and start caring for yourself.* Hazelden Publishing.
18. Solomon, M. (1994). *The power of positive dependency in intimate relationships.* Simon and Schuster.
19. Solomon, M. (1994). *Lean on me.* Simon and Schuster, p. 45.

# 2 The Sociological Failings of Codependency

## Culturally Aware Evaluation and Assessment

At every level of clinical education, training, and practice, ethical professionals must explore and incorporate a client's specific cultural beliefs, spiritual beliefs, and experience. Without obtaining the required details related to our patients' cultural backgrounds, our understanding of the client's problems, needs, and any related diagnoses can go sideways fast. Sadly, a *culturally neutral* or *culturally avoidant* client evaluation can lead to unintended consequences that can render our clinical work ineffective or even harmful. When we do not probe for a client's cultural and spiritual information, our evaluations falter, which can leave them feeling misunderstood, ignored, or diminished.

Assessments that lack cultural relevance are often founded in the mistaken belief that *most folks pretty much feel and think about the world in the same ways as we do*. This kind of thought error can lead therapists away from the accurate formation of aligned and useful diagnoses. By deeply embedding cultural curiosity into our patient's evaluations, regardless of how a client may present or act in our presence, we gain a more rounded and insightful view. Our deep, empathetic curiosity is shown when we take time to gain insight into a client's ethnic background, customs, spiritual beliefs, age, gender, and related values. By asking such questions, we not only avoid inaccurate or partial diagnoses, but we also improve our patient/provider relationship. Such considerations must be integrated at every stage of our work.

Marianne Diaz, a clinician and social justice advocate, puts it this way.

> Clinicians should anticipate that culture (as much as nature/nurture), can and will affect the decisions, beliefs, and behaviors our clients exhibit. Thus, those who seek to provide excellent clinical care should never underestimate how their client's cultural (and religious) beliefs and experiences will inform all client interactions, diagnoses, and treatment plans.[1]

To conceptualize this point, let's review some relatively minor cultural issues that might lead to misdiagnosis. In one small example, a woman walking around topless on a beach will get arrested if she is in the US, Canada, or

DOI: 10.4324/9781003058359-3

the UK. Yet partial public nudity on beaches is more or less a norm throughout much of Europe. So, how do we diagnose the German woman sent to us for therapy because she was caught and ticketed on multiple occasions for showing up topless at local beaches?

In another example, sociological research and experience with many Asian, Hispanic, African American, and Middle Eastern cultures inform us that it is often the custom for healthy heterosexual men to live with their family of origin until married. Now imagine your thoughts (from a Caucasian-American cultural perspective) when the 34-year-old Hispanic man seeking your help with dating and intimacy tells you that he has never lived independently from his mother?

Based on norms of autonomy and self-reliance that are endemic to most Western cultures, how easy would it be to pathologize either or both of the previously mentioned cases? And when clinicians lack the required cultural insights needed to provide effective client care, that is exactly what might occur.

To this point, effective clinical care requires us to ask the types of questions presented next upon initial assessment. Sadly, such questions are far too often absent from our typical evaluations, even though they can (case-by-case) prove meaningful and useful toward more effective client care.

1. To what degree do you feel your life has been affected by race/ethnicity?
2. Do you experience prejudice based on your race/ethnicity/religion? If so, please explain.
3. Do you feel more comfortable among people of your own race, culture, or ethnicity than among the general population? Why or why not?
4. Do you think that your race, ethnicity, religious beliefs, etc., affect your day-to-day life in a meaningful way? If so, how?
5. Do you ever wish you were born into a culture/ethnicity/religion other than your own?
6. Have you felt or do you feel disadvantaged in your work, family, or community related to your race, ethnicity, class, or faith?

## Effective Treatment Methods Are Cross-Cultural

The basic building blocks of all proven and effective clinical modalities must be applicable *across cultures*. We don't abandon successful models of clinical care related to culture, we build upon them, and we adapt them – provided they are adaptable.

As reflected in the previous examples, regardless of culture, race, sex, or ethnicity, clients suffering from trauma universally require modalities involving reflective, gentle forms of care (somatic, EMDR, meditation, visualization, and the like), while those with behavioral addictions require a more direct approach.

Adapting our work means utilizing the most effective forms of treatment inclusive of the client's cultural background and beliefs without abandoning the essential tenets of the chosen modality. In one example, clients whose lives are deeply rooted in Christian religious beliefs can feel mistrusting of therapies that lack an integration of biblical scripture. When working with such clients, we need to interweave validated, useful therapy methods with our client's deeply held religious beliefs or we need to refer them out to someone who can.

This doesn't mean that psychodynamic, Jungian, somatic, or any other therapy should be avoided when working with people with differing backgrounds. It does mean that the method chosen must be adapted to meet that person *where that person is*. We can pick any mode of therapy we believe will be effective with the issues presented, and then it's our job to make those concepts applicable. However, this is only possible by utilizing therapy modalities that are universally adaptable.

Eurocentric treatment models like Codependency are, by definition, grounded in concepts of personal development, self-actualization, and individuation rather than dependence on family and collective community bonds. Thus, the Codependency model at its core is inapplicable when applied to families, ethnicities, cultures, and religions that inherently value community-sourced healing over self-reliance.

Reflecting this challenge to the treatment process, Marianne Diaz states:

> As we know, acculturation has been a problem for people of color in America. For example, a lot of therapeutic processes and theories that Hispanic clients get exposed to amount to their being told that they have to "find time for themselves" or "initiate more self-care" – in other words, to individuate. This does not really resonate with the Hispanic population as we are a culture about the collective. So when you start hearing a clinician say – and it's not intentional, it's just what they know – "make time for yourself, you need not worry so much about the family," that in itself has people in my community thinking, "You don't get me and my culture." Because in the Hispanic culture, thinking that way makes you selfish.[2]

As the primary goals of Codependency are unquestionably rooted in concepts of personal growth and self-reliance over community, the model cannot be defined as cross-cultural. Any therapeutic process that skews heavily toward individual healing over leaning into the collective for support is anathema to most Native American, African American, Asian, and Hispanic cultures – to name just a few. For such people, a focus on personal growth can be viewed as selfish and in direct conflict with deeply held community-focused values. In this way, Codependency fails to meet the standards for a cross-cultural model of treatment.

## Gender Bias in Therapy

No one is immune from other's perceptions of them based on age, skin color, class, ethnicity, religious beliefs, etc. And, as stated earlier, counseling and therapy are required to incorporate such concerns in order to provide accurate and effective work. But this alone is not enough. To gain deeper, more personal insight into our patients, we must also account for gender bias.

Useful evaluations must also consider the myriad ways in which explicit and implicit gender bias affects the lives of those we treat. Gender bias and gender prejudice stem from deeply held cultural, religious, scientific, and other belief systems combined with our own imperfect perceptions of sex and gender. And gender bias is not hard to find. Consider the profound income disparities between those working in traditional female caregiving roles (teacher, counselor, mother, nurse, etc.) versus those who are toiling away in a "man's world" of business, finance, and the like. And when was the last time you heard a man complain about being catcalled on a city street by a *woman* making lewd, sexual comments?

Now consider the degree to which nearly all women experience such macro and micro aggressions daily. Almost universally, women are the most frequent targets of gender-based mistreatment and abuse, followed closely by those who demonstrate non-binary gender expression. Cisgender men are not immune are not immune from gender bias, but it is generally less overt.

The examples given previously are not new or even surprising. Yet who among us can understand how such experiences have affected our client's lived experience unless we ask? Even on our best day, gender bias may not be the first thing we consider when working with new clients, but the issue should always be on our minds, especially when counseling women and those who demonstrate non-binary forms of gender expression. That said, as long as we remain curious, empathetic, and open to our patient's ever-evolving story, initial clinical missteps can nearly always be repaired. When misaligned with a client's reality, we can readily correct course as guided by our relationship with them.

## Effective Therapy is Gender Neutral

Clinical errors based on being human are to be expected, but institutionalized treatment methods inherently inclusive of sex or gender bias are never acceptable. Consider how the therapy and counseling fields today view the treatment needs of homosexual and transgender clients versus the methods employed in the 1970s and 1980s. Such profound changes in our work have evolved in direct relationship to over a century of shifting social norms combined with more objective research.

In the past, flawed clinical research into these populations arose out of biased cultural beliefs about homosexuality, bisexuality, sexual fetishism, and transsexuality. This information, at the time reinforced by existing societal norms, pushed us to provide forms of therapeutic care that today are considered unethical. What we understood to be correct 40 to 50 years ago simply isn't. In the 21st century, we no longer view variations in gender expression, sexual identity, and sexual orientation (outside of sexual offending) as pathologies needing to be eliminated. In fact, today we view clinicians who continue to practice in these ways as offensive and unethical, thus causing their clients more harm than good.

This brings us back (again) to Codependency.

As feminist ideas filtered down into the therapy world via Codependency, women who demonstrated meaningful empathy, compassion, and dependency (especially toward men) were pathologized. As Janice Haaken stated in 1990,

"The codependency literature focuses almost exclusively on pathology, basing itself on a deficit rather than a strength-based model of women's personalities."[3] The spirit of the times simply did not leave room for women to act with empathy *and* assertiveness; they had to choose one or the other. And Codependency, with its strong messages of individuation, self-reliance, and anti-dependency (from men), served to reinforce these beliefs.

In their study of the relationships between Codependency and masculinity and femininity, George Dear and Claire Roberts state that "the gender-role measures that showed the greatest association with codependency were the socially undesirable aspects of femininity and the socially desirable aspects of masculinity."[4] Similarly, in their study of Codependency and gender-stereotyped traits, Gloria Cowan and Lynda Warren conclude that the essence of Codependency is a failure to conform to "the cultural definition of the healthy man."[5]

In the 1970s and 1980s, when Codependency was in its nascency, this new form of "pathology" (over-dependence on or enmeshment with others) was not focused toward, nor did it relate to the experience of most men. After all, men had authority, power, and hundreds of years of deference to male decision-making on their side. Men weren't watching films like *9 to 5* (a story about women fighting back against male domination in the workplace). Men were watching movies like *Top Gun* that served to support and validate their sense of power. As Anne Wilson Schaef stated in 1986, "Although men can theoretically be codependent, all the literature refers almost exclusively to women as having *the disease*."[6]

Many underlying theories behind the Codependency movement appear to be inseparable from feminist goals of that era. Sociocultural messages at the time encouraged women to empower themselves by eschewing emotional strengths reflecting empathy, compassion, and community to succeed in the real world. Attachment therapists would suggest that such therapeutic ideas led many women away from healthy relational interdependence by refocusing their attention onto self-reliance and detachment. Rather than being rewarded and appreciated as caregivers, women who chose home and hearth over independence were referred to as *unenlightened*. From the mid-1980s to this day, when a woman expresses deep empathy, love, and ongoing commitment toward an addicted or otherwise troubled man, she is likely to be viewed as *part of the problem* rather than part of the solution.

Sadly, the concept of Codependency embraces a bias *against women by women* with its incessant message that being deeply and unabashedly interdependent (as are all healthy humans) means giving away your personal power. In this way, Codependency fails to validate our natural and powerful desire (and typically feminine strength) to compassionately support and help the people we love, especially when they are in trouble.

## It's All About the Relationship

Research tells us that the greatest indicator of effective counseling is the client's relationship to the counselor. By actively evolving a relationship where the client feels the clinician's empathy and earnest desire to help, we create the type of safe, foundational emotional connection required for optimal healing.

Lacking faith and trust in one's treatment provider is a death-knell to effective work. Our patients need to like us while also believing in our sincere interes and hopes for their well-being. And this, more than any skill set or treatment methodology, is the primary indicator of a positive therapeutic outcome.

Without such a trusting clinical relationship, little progress can be expected. To this point, it is antithetical to believe that such trusting, intimate, and potentially curative relationships can be formed lacking an abiding interest and active integration of the client's sociocultural background, customs, and related personal belief systems. And Codependency, for the reasons described earlier, simply does not offer that.

## The Humanistic Revolution

From the early 1960s onward, the rapidly evolving paradigm of humanistic psychotherapy propelled the counseling field away from problem-focused models like psychoanalysis and behaviorism toward strength-based models of client care. Gone was a primary focus on what was wrong with our patients and how to fix it, replaced by a new concentration on what was working and how to improve it. As stated earlier, new counseling methods are often reflective of meaningful shifts in societal norms. Thus, the rise of humanistic psychotherapy in the early 1960s mirrored a changing culture far more focused on self-exploration and consciousness-raising than the staid intellectualism of the 1950s.

As these humanistic concepts filtered down to the counseling world, they became the foundation upon which rests many of today's most effective clinical methods. Without humanistic psychotherapy, we wouldn't have psychodrama, art therapy, mindfulness, somatic work, narrative therapies, or group therapies as we know them today. Nevertheless, despite the many meaningful clinical advances that can be traced directly to those newfound belief systems, this work also brought with it some fundamental problems that endure to this day.

Humanistic theory and the clinical work that evolved out of it unquestionably viewed *personal autonomy* and *self-reliance* as the highest and best goals of successful treatment and a life well lived. These twin individualistic themes were also mirrored in pop culture via the wildly popular personal growth and Codependency movements of that time, EST (Erhard Seminars Training) being a primary example. To put it more succinctly, the aptly named Me Generation was encouraged to view self-actualization as the primary path toward both personal fulfillment and a happy life – with a conspicuously negative view of dependent relationships.

## Codependency Is Inherently Anti-dependent

One of the defining hypotheses underlying this book is the belief that Codependency is anti-dependent rather than interdependent. To this point, we need look no further than Beattie's *Codependent No More*, which states:

Stop seeking so much approval and validation from others, we don't need the approval of everyone and anyone, we only need our own approval. We have all the same sources for happiness and making choices inside of us that others do, so find and develop your own internal supply of peace, well-being and self-esteem. *Relationships help, but they cannot be our source.*[7] [Emphasis added.]

In the 21st century, such strong messages of self-actualization *via independence* no longer define our view of mental health. For the most part, such views have been replaced by relationship-focused beliefs about human fulfillment and contentment.

Despite the immediate popularity of Codependency at the time, not all clinical professionals held the same worldview. By the early 1990s, newly minted attachment theorists were pushing back against the core theories stemming from that belief system. Dr. Marion Solomon, an early progenitor of modern attachment theory, offered up such criticisms in her foundational book, *Lean On Me: The Power of Positive Dependency in Intimate Relationships*, in which she writes:

[S]elf-sufficiency at all levels of functioning continues to be presented as the epitome of psychological health and the answer to many relationship problems.... In essence we are exhorted: "Don't depend on others to love and affirm you. Know what *you* want. Find it within yourself. Be your own best friend. Heal yourself. Only then will you be mature and ready for love."... The irony here is that *feeling secure in oneself* is built on a solid network of interdependent *relationships*.... Autonomy, self-worth, self-actualization, and self-esteem are all developed within the context of interpersonal connections.[8]

Truer words were never said!

No matter how evolved the self, all of us must lean into our healthy, ongoing dependent relationships to survive and thrive. Today, we view our capacity for relational dependency as more substantive (and foundational) than our ability to grow independently via detachment. Modern attachment theory teaches us that a primary focus on the self does not lead to healthy relationships, but rather that healthy relationship dependence is the foundation upon which our successes are grown and maintained.

Codependence, however, with its emphasis on detachment and independence (over our desire to protect and support troubled loved ones), turns us away from our basic needs to maintain and protect our meaningful attachments. In essence, the model asks us to dismiss, even devalue, our innate natural response to help a failing loved one.

The time has come for a new approach when working with loved ones of addicts. The time has come for us to view loved ones of addicts not through a lens of unresolved trauma but through a lens of interdependent attachment and intimacy. We call this new model Prodependence. Instead of viewing loved ones of addicts as inevitable victims of a traumatic past that has caught up with them and is now repeating itself in their adult lives, Prodependence views them as valiant individuals struggling to love another person even in the face of a major crisis (the addiction). This new approach – what it looks like, why it is a better option, and how we believe it can best be implemented – is the focus of the remainder of this book.

## Notes

1. The Therapist (2020). Understanding mental health stigma in Black and Hispanic/Hispanic communities: An interview with Marianne Diaz and Eric Katende. *The Therapist, 2020*, 16–19.
2. The Therapist (2020). Understanding mental health stigma in Black and Hispanic/Hispanic communities: An interview with Marianne Diaz and Eric Katende. *The Therapist, 2020*, 16–19.
3. Haaken, J. (1990). A critical analysis of the co-dependence construct. *Psychiatry, 53*(4), 396–406.
4. Dear, G. E., & Roberts, C. M. (2002). The relationships between codependency and femininity and masculinity. *Sex Roles, 46*(5), 159–165.
5. Cowan, G., & Warren, L. W. (1994). Codependency and gender-stereotyped traits. *Sex Roles, 30*(9), 631–645.
6. Schaef, A. W. (1986). *Codependence: Misunderstood-mistreated*. HarperCollins.
7. Beattie, M. (1992). *Codependent no more: How to stop controlling others and start caring for yourself*. Hazelden Publishing.
8. Solomon, M. (1994). *Lean on me: The power of positive dependency in intimate relationships*. Simon and Schuster, p. 25.

# Section 2

# Understanding Prodependence

# 3 Connection, Attachment, and Abuse

## Medical Health vs. Addiction Recovery

If your beloved spouse received a cancer diagnosis and you had two kids under the age of ten, would anyone label or judge you for doing everything possible – even to the point of giving up important parts of your life – to keep your family stable and relatively happy? If you took on two jobs, quit your exercise program, resigned from the company softball team, and stopped seeing friends to address this unexpected family crisis, would anyone in your life call you out as *enmeshed* or *enabling*? And if you went to a therapist for support, would your therapist ask you to explore the ways in which your dysfunctional childhood might be pushing you into an "unhealthy obsession" with your partner's cancer diagnosis?

Of course not. Instead, friends and family would show up on your doorstep with flowers, home-cooked meals, and sincere offers to help with childcare, shopping, yard work, and housecleaning. Meanwhile, your therapist, clergy, and employer would understand and accept that your family is having a medical crisis, that you love them, and that you must give of yourself in an extraordinary way, even if that looks a little obsessed or makes you seem a bit nutty at times. And if any of these supportive individuals felt that you were overdoing your attempts at caregiving, possibly to your own or your family's detriment, they would not chastise you. Instead, they would nudge you toward caring for yourself as well as your family while offering gentle advice about how you might care for your loved ones more effectively. They wouldn't stand back and judge you; they would lean in to help.

Unfortunately, things are very different when it comes to addiction.

In contrast to the previous story, let's say your spouse became addicted to alcohol and prescription painkillers and then lost a job because of that addiction. Let's say that because of the addiction you can no longer trust your partner to adequately care for your kids. What happens now when you take that second job, stop going to the gym, stop hanging out with friends, eliminate your recreational activities, and start to obsess about your partner's problem, all the while paying the family bills and caring for your children? Will your friends and family, employer, clergy, and therapist

DOI: 10.4324/9781003058359-5

support this degree of caregiving while empathizing with your frustration and exhaustion?

Most likely they will not.

In the addiction world, support and therapy for a loving spouse (or parent) typically involves judgmental head-shaking, tut-tuts, and expressions of concern about *the caretaker's problem*, with that problem being identified as dysfunctional attempts to love, save, rescue, and heal the addict and the family.

Move over empathy; make way for judgment.

If your response to a loved one who has a serious medical disorder is to put aside your own recreation, work, or even healthy self-care, you are seen as an angel or saint. If you choose to put a medically ill person's needs over your own until they get better, you will be celebrated and supported.

But if your response to a loved one who has a serious *addictive* illness is to put aside your own recreation, work, or even healthy self-care, you are seen as enmeshed, enabling, boundary-less, controlling, and most of all – ugh – Codependent. In such cases, you'll be told that your efforts to love and care for the addict and your family are misguided and *keeping everyone stuck in the problem*. You might also be told that you need to get out of your "disease" by pulling back from all that unhealthy rescuing.

## Our Need for Connection

Humans are pack animals. We are meant to work together, not to go it alone. For evidence, think back to prehistoric times when we lived in tribes. If we went hunting, we went in a group; otherwise, we were as likely to be eaten as to eat. And hunting trips could take a long time, so other members of the tribe stayed behind and tanned hides to keep the group warm, gathered nuts and berries to eat, collected sticks for the fire, protected the vulnerable, and did some rudimentary farming.

For thousands of years, this type of communal living was the standard for survival. Because of this, our brains evolved in ways that encourage interpersonal bonding, and now *we are evolutionarily wired to be dependent* upon others. We enter the world completely reliant on other people for shelter, nutrition, and emotional support (love), and these core requirements *do not change* as we grow older. What keeps us healthy as children also keeps us healthy as adults. Even in late adolescence, when we tend to individuate from our families, we don't move toward isolation. Instead, our dependency needs shift from parents and family to peers and eventually to romantic partners.

Yet somehow, as we move into adulthood, our intrinsic need for emotional connection gets discounted. This despite the well-researched fact that people who spend their lives "apart from" rather than "a part of" do not function as well as those who feel emotionally connected.

An immense amount of mental and physical health research shows that isolated/separated individuals suffer both emotionally and physically.[1] Conversely, people who place a high value on developing and maintaining meaningful connections tend to be happier, more resilient, and more successful.[2]

They even tend to live longer.[3] Thus, we see that emotionally intimate connections are nearly as essential to life and well-being as more obvious needs like food, water, and shelter. Without healthy dependency and connection, we may make it physically, but we won't be happy. When we go it alone, we fail to thrive. And this deeply ingrained need for emotional connection does not abate simply because a person with whom we feel an intimate bond is challenged by an addiction or some other serious issue.

Consider, for instance, a study of married couples where one partner was told that, while in a brain scanner, they were going to receive an electric shock on the ankle every time an X appeared on a video screen visible in the scanner. When in the scanner alone, the "danger zones" of these individuals' brains lit up like crazy. The same was true when a doctor or nurse held their hand to comfort them. When their spouse held their hand, however, their neurobiological threat response calmed significantly. Moreover, the level of calming was directly influenced by the quality of the participant's marriage. Those with happy marriages were more easily soothed by their partner, and vice versa.[4]

Other studies also support the need for healthy connection. For example:

- A consistent sense of loneliness can raise blood pressure to the point where the risk of heart attack and stroke doubles.[5]
- Distress in an existing relationship increases the risk of heart problems.[6]
- Distress in an existing relationship increases the risk of problems with the immune and hormonal systems.[7]
- Social isolation and relationship distress have been thought to lead to the common cold.[8]
- Social isolation and relationship distress have been linked to lowered odds of surviving a natural disaster.[9]

The research goes on and on, repeatedly revealing an undeniable link between a lack of healthy connections and diminished well-being. One study suggests that this link is every bit as strong and every bit as damning as the link between smoking and poor health.[10] When we feel securely attached to trusted others, we are healthier, we are more confident, we take more healthy risks, we reach our career goals faster, and we are more willing to explore and take advantage of life opportunities (of all types).[11] Stated very simply, we do better in all aspects of life when we feel loved and supported. When we feel securely connected, we blossom and grow.

So how can emotional dependence be a weakness?

Dr. Sue Johnson states the matter as succinctly and eloquently as anyone, writing, "Love is not the icing on the cake of life. It is a basic primary need, like oxygen or water."[12] We need to hold one another, we need to care for one another in healthy ways, and we need to overtly express our love and have that love returned. Without this, we suffer. Just as we would if we were not eating or sleeping. And this truth does not diminish because we are dealing with a loved one's addiction.

## Addicts and the Need for Connection

Addicts need intimate connection as much as if not more than most people. An all-time great illustration of this occurs in Canadian researcher Bruce Alexander's famed "Rat Park" study. Prior to Alexander's work, it was generally believed that pleasure, as wrought by addictive substances and behaviors, was the primary driver of addiction. Bolstering this belief was the fact that most early research on the root causes of addiction centered on the neurochemical pleasure response, and on the fact that lab rats, when given the choice, would almost always choose to drink opiate-infused water over regular water. For a long while, even the National Institute on Drug Abuse espoused this "pleasure drives addiction" viewpoint.[13]

However, based solely on the fact that most people do not become addicts (for instance, the Substance Abuse and Mental Health Services Administration estimates that almost every American adult has tried alcohol, but only about 6.8% become alcoholic[14]), it seemed clear to at least a few addiction treatment specialists and researchers that pleasure was *not* the primary driver of addiction, that the desire for pleasure was *not* what caused some (but not all) people (and rats) to return to a potentially addictive substance or behavior over and over, compulsively and to their detriment.

Recognizing this, Alexander reexamined the results of then-existing rat studies, where test subjects were placed in empty cages, alone, with two water bottles to choose from – one with pure water, the other with opiate-infused water. In those experiments, the rats uniformly got hooked on and eventually overdosed on the opiate water, leading researchers to conclude that the out-of-control search for extreme pleasure drives addictions. This led to a belief that addicts were just weak people, and if they could only develop some willpower, things would be OK.

Alexander disagreed. He was bothered by the fact that the cages in which lab rats were isolated were small, with no potential for stimulation beyond the opiate water. He thought, "Of course they get high. What else are they supposed to do?" In response, he created the rat park, a cage approximately 200 times larger than the typical isolation cage, with hamster wheels and multicolored balls to play with, plenty of tasty food to eat, and spaces for mating and raising litters.[15] And he put not one rat but 20 rats (of both genders) into the cage. Then, and only then, did he mirror the old experiments.

## Rat Love

And guess what? Alexander's rats ignored the opiate water, expressing much more interest in typical communal rat activities such as playing, fighting, eating, and mating. Even rats who'd previously been isolated and drinking the drugged water left it alone when they were placed in the rat park. With a little bit of social stimulation and connection, addiction in rats disappeared.

Happily, this result transfers to humans, though in somewhat more complicated ways. With proper direction, support, and a fair amount of conscious effort, individuals who were not graced with secure childhood attachments (and therefore the ability to easily and comfortably connect in adulthood) can develop earned security via long-term therapy, 12-step groups, and various other healthy and healing relationships – *the most important of which are healthy connections with loved ones.*

Interestingly, addiction treatment specialists and the 12-step community have unconsciously operated with this principle in mind for decades. In fact, much of what occurs in well-informed, group-focused addiction treatment programs and 12-step recovery (beyond breaking through the addict's denial and putting a stop to the addictive behavior) is geared, either directly or indirectly, toward the development of reliably healthy social bonds.

That said, developing healthy intimate connections can be difficult, especially for addicts, who nearly always have histories of chronic childhood trauma and other forms of early-life dysfunction that can make intimate, adult attachments uncomfortable and difficult. For addicts, learning to trust, reducing shame, and feeling comfortable with emotional and social vulnerability takes time, ongoing effort, and a knowledgeable, willing, and empathetic support network (therapists, fellow recovering addicts, friends, employers, and, of course, *intimately connected loved ones*).

## Connection vs. Independence

No matter how evolved the self, all of us must lean into healthy, ongoing dependent relationships to survive and thrive. In the 21st century, as we are now profoundly influenced by attachment theory, we view our relational dependencies as more substantive than our ability to grow independently via detachment. We now believe that a primary focus on the self does not encourage interdependence but instead leads us toward anti-dependence and narcissism.

Codependence, with its emphasis on self-reflection and independence (over connecting with and relying on others), asks us to turn away from our basic need for an enduring lifeline of connection to others. This although even the most independent among us secretly (sometimes unconsciously) longs for deep engagement and shared dependence.

Twenty-first century evaluations and therapies are no longer solely focused on individual functioning. Instead, they consider the ways that our clients' lives are supported by others. Although it seems like a given today, it is only in the past few decades that the counseling field has arrived at the understanding that human beings are happier and more effective when working through life's painful challenges together and that by sharing our joys and losses with intimate friends, family, and community, our lives take on deeper meaning.

## Attachment Matters

So many experiences, activities, and interactions drive our ability to form and maintain meaningful relationships. The interactive call and response of mother and child is at the start of the process, later followed by familial, social, peer, community, and ultimately spouse and family bonds. And yet there is one quality that both encompasses and is the foundation for health attachments at any age, and that quality is trust. Without relational reliability, consistency, and an environment where the needs of the child come before those of the caregiver, trust is not established. Other issues in our relationships may lead us to varied emotional and intellectual responses to those experiences, but healthy people who attach in caring responsive ways throughout their lifetimes get there via nature and nurture. The nature part is simply who we are – personality, reactivity, self-regulation, and all the rest that lead to our naturally being more open or more self-protective. In other words, we can be fairly certain that we come out of the womb either more or less equipped for social bonding. Once we are born (perhaps prior), nurture then takes over by layering our relational interactive experiences on top of our natural bonding abilities.

Current writers and researchers in the field of attachment continue to enrich our understanding of how to best treat those with disruptions and injuries to their primary relationships that can lead to adult addictions. For example, Dr. Stan Tatkin identifies such situations as potential "deal breakers," as a secure-functioning relationship requires mutual trust, transparency with information, and the ability to create safety by protecting one another. He also believes a loved one who is altered by addictive behaviors will become unavailable – emotionally, mentally, and physically, which can lead to feelings of neglect and abandonment in the partner.[16] Anyone living with addiction knows that one of the primary challenges for addicts is the ability to be honest, thereby creating trust and safety. Where there is no trust, there can be no intimacy or secure attachment.

As Prodependence treatment is focused on effective relational dependency, it is relevant to note that newer research challenges the notion of human dependency within relationships as being negative. In fact, Levine and Heller contend that the more effective the dependency between individuals, the more autonomous they can become within that relationship.[17] This underscores earlier research that focused on the importance of a secure base from which effectively dependent individuals can take more risk and live life more freely, because they know their significant other is consistent, reliable, and safe. Because humans have this proclivity to create and sustain bonds with others, individuals within intimate relationships each rely on that relationship to provide affection, closeness, comfort, and security, ideally creating deep psychological and physiological interdependence.[18] This secure sense of interdependence is necessary for these relationships to sustain and maintain the delicate balance of both autonomy and connection.

In addition to human bonding, the inclination to care for significant others is also a biologically wired phenomenon. It is nonsensical to suggest that the desire and need to do this is based in some other internal pathology; however, Prodependence does not subscribe to relational caretaking and helping at the expense or to the detriment of the caretaker. A balanced approach of maintaining personal safety while navigating the tumultuous waves of attachment injuries is always at the forefront of treatment.

## Attachment Styles

Adult attachment styles generally refer to way in which individuals connect (or do not connect) throughout the life span, beginning with their earliest relationships. Levine and Heller (2019)[19] point out that understanding the four attachment styles (secure, anxious-ambivalent, disorganized, and avoidant) – or a combination of them – can assist a therapist in predicting behavior in their adult relationships. Although the Prodependence model is heavily based on attachment theories, specifically regarding human connection within the construct of relationships where the issue of addiction is present, it does not focus on *attachment styles*. The authors' discussions of *attachment* used throughout this book refer to the human neurobiological propensity for intimate and secure human bonding. A foundational belief of Codependence is those who remain by the side of an active addict do so because they are similarly *troubled* themselves. A foundational belief of Prodependence is those who remain by the side of an active addict do so because they are deeply and meaningfully *attached* to that person.

## The Neurochemistry of Attachment

The early stages of attachment and falling in love in a romantic relationship not only include the genetic predisposition for bonding, but it also involves a literal chemical reaction. Specific naturally occurring chemicals in the brain such as norepinephrine and oxytocin are present, contributing to the bonding experience and desire to remain securely connected. Shorter lived chemicals such as norepinephrine are present during the infatuation or limerence stage, while oxytocin – a more persistent chemical – contributes to long-term attachment and bonding.[20] This understanding can aid the clinician in understanding the traumatic nature of betrayal or disconnection in these relationships.

The interpersonal injuries caused by addictive behaviors, or attachment ruptures, indicate that something external has broken or threatened to destroy the delicate threads of connection holding two individuals together. Addictive behaviors will compete with the understandable need for the attention and care of the individual engaging in them. This will sound the alarm of the partner or loved one, usually initiating desperate attempts to hold the connection together by any means necessary. Prodependence understands these are not indicators of a crazy, sick, or unhealthy individual – rather a literal, raging chemical and physiological firestorm that demands immediate attention.

## Interdependence and Attachment

Trusting, interdependent relationships evolve over time as we learn to lean into our own *and* our loved one's strengths, while simultaneously accepting and honoring our individual vulnerabilities and shared emotional needs. This path toward deepening levels of relational intimacy and healthy dependency is established via a consistent aligned commitment to open communication, mutual learning, and integrity. In simpler terms, *healthy* loved ones grow toward one another, by learning that they are safe to express their own needs, while also being willing and able to support those of the other and vice versa. If successfully executed, the stable family unit that grows from this process tends to create its own unique, systemic process that is both invitational to the outside world *and* protective from it. The development of these healthy individual and group dynamics can be thwarted if any of the individuals involved are emotionally challenged to accept and be adaptive to changing relational dynamics. While overly rigid boundaries tend to stagnate and distance a couple-ship, overly enmeshed relationships put unnecessary (often unconscious) limits on intimacy, sexuality, and the open expression of difficult feelings. Finding a tolerable and effective balance of these two ends of the emotional spectrum is a big part of the journey toward creating a foundation of respectful, long-term loving relationships.

## Abuse and Addiction Are Intertwined

Actively addicted and newly sober people, impaired by their own denial, shame, and narcissism, are often emotionally reactive and volatile, especially toward those closest to them. This is especially true if the addict is still using or acting out. Insults are thrown, sometimes accompanied by plates or fists, doors slammed, threats made, and things said in front of children that cannot be unsaid. Most often at the receiving end of this drama are angry, hurting, and overwhelmed family, spouses, and the friends who, more often than not, get blamed for this addiction-fueled craziness. Sober or not, addicted people *by definition* struggle to avoid impulsive, emotionally driven decision-making. This often leads to them acting out strongly felt emotions, rather than seeking healthy, more engaged solutions.

But it is not just the addict who can become emotionally reactive, raging, and withdrawn. In a weak moment, beloved spouses, friends, and family may also act in ways later they regret. As one wife recently reported in group therapy,

> Sometimes I got so furious when he would come home drunk that I would hit him. Several times the authorities were called to our home, not because of my addicted husband, but because of me. I'm so ashamed. I mean, I always knew that he was deeply troubled and broken, but that didn't keep me from flying off the handle. Looking back, I see that over time I became someone I never thought I would be, someone who is angry and abusive just like him.

## Abuse Thrives Behind Closed Doors

It's a sad truth that emotional trauma and physical abuse more often than not remain hidden behind the scenes in troubled family relationships where addiction is present. Typically, spouses, parents, close friends, even the addicts themselves will hide such realities from outsiders fearing shame, judgment, or being seen as *that family*. In some situations, slapping, screaming, shoving, and breaking things to show upset are not viewed as "real abuse." Others fear the consequences of adult or child mistreatment becoming known to child welfare, the police, or other authorities, so they will say and do nothing.

Unfortunately, clinical research tells us that many abuse survivors will adapt to being mistreated by slowly beginning to view such experiences as *deserved* or as a *new normal* (learned helplessness). They too will say and do nothing.

Most families with abusive dynamics will close ranks and hide these problems in the service of maintaining a *looking good* exterior. Thus, adult *and child* mistreatment of various sorts frequently goes underreported or unreported in such circumstances. Sadly, as closed family systems are subject to entropy, previously loving, supportive, and intimate relationships can degrade into frustrating disconnection, verbal or physical threats, shaming, humiliation, and violence. As problematic compulsive behaviors and substance use escalate, so does the emotional volatility of addicts and those who love them.

## Addicts Get Abused Too

There is not a partner or close family member of any active addict not filled regularly with rage, sadness, and disappointment. After all, who wouldn't feel impotent, powerless, and paralyzed in such situations? Just as no one in relationship with an addict should stay around for abuse or threats, no addict (despite their history) should stay around for meaningful abuse or threats from those who care about them – even if they think they deserve it (and they often think they do). One addict put it this way:

> After all I put her though, I can understand her wanting to cause me pain because I deserve it. So, when she yells or hits me or even walks out with the kids, I just let it go. Why should I expect anything better after all the years I've been using drugs and hurting her? After all, I have enough trouble trying to keep her from just leaving me, so a few bruises, threats, or broken plates are the least of my problems.

There are times or situations in which addicts must put their own physical and emotional self-care and survival over their relationships – at least for a period of time. Sometimes this means that an addict must call out for help or create a safety list and an escape plan. Whatever our clinical perspective, Prodependent or not, when treating anyone closely associated with addiction (regardless of whether they are a loved one, spouse, couple, family, or addict), our clinical work is inadequate and incomplete without a thorough exploration and inventory of all forms of potential abuse.

All of us have faced angry, dysregulated clients whose life experiences have left them saying things and acting in ways that are unhelpful, even harmful.

Some are reacting to past issues evoked by current circumstances (regression), while others are simply trying to get by after years of unresolved addictive behavior. Ultimately, it doesn't matter how hurt or angry one feels in such circumstances, abusing and threatening other people can never effect positive change. At the same time, it leaves behind it a legacy of long-term pain and disconnection. *The potential for many forms of mistreatment to become activated in relationships dealing with addiction is high.* Thus, all addiction and mental health professionals clinically involved with such cases should evaluate for verbal, emotional, and physical abuse so we can intervene if required.

## Typical Abuse Scenarios

While it is beyond the scope of this text to review all forms of abuse and their effects, the authors feel it is important to touch on a few of the primary types of abuse that tend to be a hallmark of relationships and families with addicted loved ones. The following headings and lists are meant to be an overview of differing types of maltreatment. A more extensive and thorough abuse assessment tool – *which the authors strongly encourage be used* – can be found at the end of this chapter. It was not our intention to cover every major area of this topic; thus, we advise using this information as a jumping off point toward obtaining a more detailed assessment via the evaluation at the end of this chapter.

## Externalization and Gaslighting

This is an attempt to deny a loved one's reality and intuition. This leads them to question reality as they see it, thereby creating emotional confusion, self-doubt, and internal distress. This is a form of manipulation meant to shift responsibility for the addiction from the addict to others around them.

## Abuse of Loved Ones via Externalization

- Telling or implying that they drink, use, or act out *because* their loved ones are expressing anger, upset, or sorrow about the addiction.
- Baldfaced lying when facing inconvenient truths (gaslighting).
- Telling others that they drink, use, and act out *because of them.*
- Playing the victim to manipulate and distract others into feeling compassion and empathy rather than concern. Example: "I had so much trauma when I was a kid, why do you give me a hard time about drinking when you know what I went through."
- Telling others that they are "making a big deal out of nothing."

## Emotional Abuse

This is a way to control another person by emotionally challenging, criticizing, embarrassing, shaming, blaming, or otherwise manipulating another person.

Basic signs of emotional abuse include:

- Hypercritical, consistently judgmental.
- Ignoring boundaries, invading privacy, sharing secrets.
- Frequently dismissing or disregarding the other's feelings and beliefs.
- Being possessive and/or controlling of the other.
- Manipulation via fear by threatening abandonment, abuse, or both.
- Repeatedly arguing and challenging intimate others to believe that what they see or what they remember is not true (invalidating another's reality or gaslighting).
- Devaluing another's value, worth, looks, feelings, thoughts, and beliefs.

## Physical Abuse

This can be defined as any non-accidental physical injury to another person and can include striking, kicking, burning, shoving, biting, or any type of behavior that results in physical harm or impairment.

Basic signs of physical abuse include:

- Black eyes and bruises.
- Split or bloody lips.
- Red or purple marks on the neck, hands, and back.
- Sprained wrists, arms, and shoulders.
- Broken bones and sprains.
- A typical use of heavy make-up or clothes that cover the entire body to hide injuries.

Many forms of verbal and emotional abuse – while uncomfortable, hurtful, sad, and even scary – at times do not necessarily require a client to plan to leave, but rather to plan how to stay connected to and supported by others who can be relied on for emotional support and safety.

## Sexual Abuse

This can be defined as sexual comments, language, and/or behavior that is undesired, nonconsensual, and, in many cases, illegal.

Sexual abuse is on a continuum from no-touch offenses like inappropriate and sexually offensive comments in the office all the way to rape and other forms of sexual violence. Sexual abuse is always inclusive of unwanted sexual contact or threats. Sexual assault occurs when someone touches any part of another person's body in a sexual way, even on top of clothing, without that person's consent (including if the other person is not old enough or healthy enough to consent). Such abuse can take place within the context of an intimate or marital relationship. When working with such cases, it is essential for us to inquire about a couple's or loved one's sexuality to promote awareness and safety where required.

Basic forms of familial sexual abuse include:

- Incest and/or child abuse.
- Exposing/introducing children (or vulnerable adults) to pornography, sexual situations, cheating, and the like.
- Leaving porn or sexual content around for children to find.
- Letting children know about or view parental infidelity and cheating.
- Bringing new or unknown sex partners into a home where children reside.
- Forcing partners or others to have sex without their consent.
- Sexualizing or negatively shaming a child's sexual and physical development.
- Shaming or devaluing another's body or sexual expression.
- Homophobia, transphobia.
- Inviting spouses into unwanted sexual situations, that is, group sex, threesomes, etc.

As with physical and emotional abuse previously mentioned, no one should tolerate any form of sexual abuse, especially in a beloved partnership or marriage. Such cases should be identified and a client safety plan put into place.

---

**About Betrayal**

When cheating is discovered (romantic or sexual), the betrayed partners are nearly always emotionally traumatized. Even if they suspected that something was amiss in the relationship before discovering the problem, even if the infidelities are purely drug and alcohol related, they will nonetheless be deeply wounded when learning the truth. Those who learn about cheating by an intimate partner typically experience stress and anxiety symptoms characteristic of post-traumatic stress disorder. PTSD is a very serious, potentially life-threatening problem – a psychological reaction to an especially traumatic event. The symptoms commonly include flashbacks, nightmares, severe anxiety, hypervigilance, and powerful mood swings (including flashes of extreme anger, insecurity, and/or fear). This type of reactivity will continue until the sexual or romantic acting out has stopped or there is a meaningful end to the committed relationship. In such situations, it is highly unlikely that an active addict will be able to commit to relational or sexual behavior change. Without prior elimination of substance abuse and alcoholism, behavioral problems are nearly impossible to treat, as the substances themselves disinhibit the addict's motivation and ability *to just say no* (to gaming, gambling, spending, porn, and the like) and make better choices.

## Familial Abuse

Abuse appears in the family when the basic needs of children, elders, and other dependent individuals are unmet, denied, or abused. Exposure of vulnerable individuals to violence, verbal abuse, splitting, neglect, threats of violence, devaluing, shaming, and dismissing needs counts as familial abuse.

Examples of familial abuse include:

- Removing children from the home without informing other caregivers.
- Splitting parental relationships by pitting one parent against the other (children).
- Insecurity – holding children or others to unattainable standards, then treating them as inferior when they fail.
- Narcissistic parenting – where the needs of the adult exceed the needs of the child, thereby making the child feel guilty for putting their own needs above those of the parent.
- Hostility and rejection – withholding love and affection, blaming and shaming family members over minor issues, threatening rejection and/or abandonment.
- Leaving children unsafe – driving drunk, not picking them up at school, etc. Fighting, arguing, throwing, hitting, and the like – with children present.

Prodependent tools to help loved ones who are being abused by the addict include:

- Educating, exploring, and growing client awareness of what defines abuse – verbal and physical.
- Avoiding engagement when the addict is being abusive by taking "time outs" and knowing when/how to leave.
- Helping loved ones create and maintain healthy boundaries.
- Building a support network of healthy others who are already aware of what is going on in the family/friendship.
- Creating an exit plan.
- Ensuring financial and other safety by consulting an attorney or online site related to potential financial abuse or legal actions.

## Creating a Safety Plan

When there has been actual or inferences of potential physical abuse like pushing, shoving, hitting, slapping, physically blocking the other from leaving, holding them down, threatening violence, yelling, emotional withdrawal, blaming, shaming, threatening abandonment, and the like, we must work with our clients to develop a safety plan.

Possible elements of a *safety plan* include:

- Identifying a safe friend or friends and safe places to go.
- Keeping an alternate cellphone nearby.

- Memorizing the phone numbers of friends, family, or shelters.
- Making a list of things to take if leaving quickly.
- Getting educated about all the aspects of abusive relationships.
- Hiding an extra set of car keys.
  Doing a "fire drill" alone or with kids to practice leaving if needed.
- Ensuring that at least one safe person knows exactly what is going on.
- Asking the doctor how to get extra medicine or medically necessary items.
- Protecting self in online security and social media.
- Trying to take any evidence of abuse or violence.
- Keeping copies of paper and electronic documents, financial and bank information on an external thumb drive or in the cloud for ready access if needed.

## Abuse and the Codependency Model

Although the Codependency model does not condone abuse of any kind, the perspective focuses heavily on the deficits and "pathology" of the partner and may have the unintended impact of giving the addict *additional* reasons to blame, be unkind, or even abusive to the partner. In a way, it can provide the addict a way out of taking responsibility for their behavior, as it offers them additional reasons and justifications to use. It also heavily encourages partners or loved ones toward autonomy and disconnection from the addict, thus promoting an environment where abuse can grow and thrive (as less connection may feel like *less accountability* to an active addict).

Unfortunately, these perspectives have been pervasive in the therapeutic world since the early days of treating spouses of alcoholics in the 1940s and 1950s. Addiction historian William White (2005) suggests that due to their overt expressions of distress, wives of alcoholics were perceived in this way: the general view of the alcoholic wife depicted in the early AA and psychotherapy literature was that of a woman who was neurotic, sexually repressed, dependent, man-hating, domineering, mothering, guilty and masochistic, and/or hostile and nagging.

The typical therapist's view of the wife of an alcoholic at that time generally was one of "I'd drink too, if I were married to her." When seen from this perspective, Codependence can simply be considered as a newer, more sophisticated form of the victim shaming that has been endemic in our views of the loved ones of addicts from day one.

## Abuse and the Prodependence Model

The Prodependence model addresses abuse by seeking to understand and confront the negative and harmful behavior using whatever tools necessary toward establishing personal and familial safety. Unlike the Codependency model that would encourage the loved one to focus primarily on their part in the problem and completely detach from the addict for safety, Prodependence sees the abusive behavior for what it is: Abusive behavior.

Prodependence does not require that anyone *take responsibility* for another's abuse, although the tendency of most abusive people is to externalize the source of their anger. Rather, the model asks us to work toward identification and elimination from the very start, rather than any focus on insight. Abuse in any form, by anyone involved, must be the primary focus of the clinical work until all parties are guaranteed physical and emotional safety, regardless of how this is achieved.

In summary, Prodependence:

- Acknowledges the reality and effects of abuse within the relationship.
- Focuses on the source of a loved one's distress.
- Celebrates a desire for safe and meaningful connection.
- Recognizes the distress of loved ones as a trauma response.
- Encourages safe attachment when/where/if possible.

---

### Prodependence Does Not Mean Living with Abuse

Prodependence holds no tolerance for abuse, even though the model does not encourage overall detachment. However, without question, Prodependence, as does any ethical and effective treatment model, strongly encourages self-preservation on every level. We seek all the information we can gather in our evaluations, later utilizing this information to help clients create an appropriate and useful safety plan. Prodependence is fully focused on helping troubled people find deeper connection, meaning, and healing through their relationships, but never at the cost of one's health, safety, well-being, or sanity. Sometimes, the most loving and supportive thing to do is to withdraw, especially when personal safety is of primary concern.

---

## Remain Involved or Let Them Go?

### *For the Partner*

A dilemma with which partners of addicts frequently wrestle is whether they should stay or leave a relationship. First and foremost, the decision to remain in or exit a relationship is a personal choice. There is no scenario in which we – the therapist – should make that choice for a client; however, we do have to responsibility to help the client navigate the injuries to the relationship while simultaneously considering and evaluating the client's safety. This can be challenging as each client's specific needs for safety may differ. When experiencing waves of grief due to the uncontrolled losses in their relationship, a partner usually develops understandable questions about the situation and the addict in their life.

- Will they ever have my back?
- Will they be there for me?
- Will they ever understand what they have put me through?

- Can I ever trust them again?
- How can I keep from worrying that they will drink again?
- How can I get angry when they blame the drinking on our conflicts?

There are situations that may obviously require physical distance for safety (see section on abuse), and then there are those that may not be so apparent. Just like each vessel on the water has a unique Plimsoll line that determines how much load weight it can handle before taking on water and sinking (Thomas, 1989); so do partners have their own "internal Plimsoll line" that determines their individual limit for what they can manage in the relationship. Assisting the clients navigating their own limits throughout their sojourn will be very useful, even if that means the clients may need to leave the relationship for their own well-being.

The following are examples of situations in which partners and/or family may choose to stay to provide ongoing support to the addict. Remaining emotionally and physically close to an addict who is using or newly sober requires that the addict is:

- Not being abusive.
- Actively seeking help and intervention for themselves.
- Being honest and transparent.
- Is aware that their addictive problems are theirs to fix and not the fault of parents, partners, and the like.
- Is taking responsibility for their actions and decisions.
- Has moments of empathy and compassion for people and situations in which they have caused harm.
- Initiating and maintaining their own recovery-self-care (12-step meetings, therapies etc.) without having to be nagged, begged, or pushed into doing the right thing.

Examples of situations in which partners may choose (or need) to leave include:

- They no longer want to help or support the addict.
- They no longer wish to remain in the relationship.
- A lack of physical or emotional safety.
- When there are emotional, physical, financial, sexual, or other forms of active abuse.
- The addict remains in denial and unwilling to consider addressing the addiction.
- The addict continues cycles of abuse with partner and/or other loved ones.
- The addict refuses to be honest and transparent.
- The addict's behavior leaves family, loved ones, or spouse in an endless cycle of blame and chaos.
- The addict is causing harm to family – children, parents, siblings, etc.

### When Love Hurts – It May Be Time to Go

Prodependence does not espouse the idea that partners or family should stay in an intimate relationship with an addicted loved one simply because they naturally desire to remain attached and bonded. Instead, Prodependence acknowledges the healthy desire to remain closely connected even if remaining attached to their current partner is no longer a safe and viable option. Prodependence teaches how to push the addictive relationship aside for survival and stability, fully knowing those actions may or may not influence change in the addict. Prodependence helps to manage, tolerate, and influence the relationship with the addict, thereby supporting self and the addict's healing/recovery without pathologizing the desire to healthfully remain closely aligned with the troubled loved one. However, other than evident safety issues that will require separation, the Prodependence model suggests that larger permanent decisions about staying or leaving the relationship be delayed until the crisis has passed or the client has achieved greater emotional and physical stability. Possible feedback from the therapist might be, "It's okay to not decide what you should do now, let's take it one day at a time."

### For Parents, Siblings, Children, and Others Who Are Closely Related to the Addict

For the loved ones or family members of addicts, the decision about when to help and when to leave them (or ask them to leave) is never easy. These decisions typically come with a plethora of directly related considerations such as the addicts':

- Age.
- Type and/or style of addiction.
- Mental, physical, and emotional stability.
- Addictive and mental health history – past relapses, going off prescribed medication, not attending health care and other self-care appointments.
- Willingness to engage and seek help.
- Financial and other resources.
- Physical and emotional health.

Although these are very personal choices, based on many different factors, we should in no way assign pathology or shame to the decision to stay or go, to support or not, etc. We need to consider all circumstances while aiding all loved ones in figuring out the correct path for them. This includes not only what is best not only for the addict, but for everyone involved.

### Addiction in the Family (Non-spousal)

Example: Married parents have an adult son who is addicted to drugs. They have spent several years and a lot of money for various therapies, in-patient treatments, housing, etc. – in the service of trying to help their child, only to find themselves without the financial or other resources to take care of themselves. Such families can lack the emotional reserves required to continue to help at this level without sacrificing their own physical and emotional well-being. The best assistance a Prodependence-based therapist may be able offer at this point is to help establish life-preserving boundaries along with sound self-care practices without inducing shame and defensiveness by pointing all the "sick" or "unhealthy" things they have done to try and save a failing son.

Prodependence acknowledges these are not easy choices, and there is rarely a single correct choice, but the desire to assist those they love does not indicate an illness or pathology. To tell a parent not to help or to detach from and abandon their addict child, or to tell an adult child to refuse to help a failing parent, is essentially telling them to not be human and ignore their natural inclinations to assist where they can and preserve the ones they love. Family members and loved ones may need to limit contact with their addicted child or reduce the amount of financial assistance they offer, but this does not mean they will ever limit or reduce the love and concern they feel as that is hard-wired into their DNA.

## APPENDIX A

### Abusive Behavior Inventory

Using a global inventory of abusive behavior (see next) can help give permission for clients to openly discuss these shameful and hurtful experiences, while offering the clinician highly useful information. Note here that the authors have *intentionally* not provided a key or related means of determining the degree of abusive behavior in a numeral form; therefore, no formal scoring instrument has been placed. This is purposeful as the goal here is not to obtain a verifiable, validated numerical gauge of abusive behavior, but rather to use this instrument as a springboard for client/therapist discussion. The inventory can also be used directly with the addict to better evaluate if they too are being abused by an overwhelmed, "out of control" spouse or family member. This is the type of essential information that clinicians need to evaluate early in treatment to both ensure safety and to devise an accurate, individualized treatment plan.

This inventory is best not sent home with the client as it can produce more discomfort than insight when reviewed alone. The inventory is best utilized during sessions as introduced and discussed question by question. The inventory can also be utilized to evaluate the responses of two separate clients side by side. This can be useful toward comparing and contrasting details of how abusive behavior plays out for the addict and for loved ones/spouses.

## ABUSIVE BEHAVIOR INVENTORY

| Client No. 1 | | Client No. 2 | | |
|---|---|---|---|---|
| **Past** | **Now** | **Past** | **Now** | |
| | | | | **PHYSICAL ABUSE** |
| ___ | ___ | ___ | ___ | Block the way, stand in doorway |
| ___ | ___ | ___ | ___ | Hold captive, keep from leaving the house |
| ___ | ___ | ___ | ___ | Lock out of shared home |
| ___ | ___ | ___ | ___ | Refuse to help sick, injured, or pregnant partner |
| ___ | ___ | ___ | ___ | Abandon partner in a dangerous place |
| ___ | ___ | ___ | ___ | Push or shove |
| ___ | ___ | ___ | ___ | Grab or hold |
| ___ | ___ | ___ | ___ | Pin to floor, bed, wall |
| ___ | ___ | ___ | ___ | Throw down or knock down |
| ___ | ___ | ___ | ___ | Slap |
| ___ | ___ | ___ | ___ | Hit with fist |
| ___ | ___ | ___ | ___ | Twist arm |
| ___ | ___ | ___ | ___ | Pull hair |
| ___ | ___ | ___ | ___ | Kick |
| ___ | ___ | ___ | ___ | Bite |
| ___ | ___ | ___ | ___ | Pinch |
| ___ | ___ | ___ | ___ | Pull hair |
| ___ | ___ | ___ | ___ | Butt heads |
| ___ | ___ | ___ | ___ | Choke, put hands to throat |
| ___ | ___ | ___ | ___ | Throw objects at partner |
| ___ | ___ | ___ | ___ | Hit with an object |
| ___ | ___ | ___ | ___ | Hit, shove, or kick pregnant partner |
| ___ | ___ | ___ | ___ | Use a weapon to hurt or threaten |
| ___ | ___ | ___ | ___ | Cause bruises, cuts, black eyes |
| ___ | ___ | ___ | ___ | Cause broken bones |
| ___ | ___ | ___ | ___ | Cause impaired vision or hearing |
| ___ | ___ | ___ | ___ | Burn or scald |
| ___ | ___ | ___ | ___ | Cause hospitalization |
| ___ | ___ | ___ | ___ | Injure or disfigure permanently |
| ___ | ___ | ___ | ___ | Prevent from receiving medical care |
| ___ | ___ | ___ | ___ | Kill or attempt to kill |
| | | | | **VERBAL ABUSE** |
| ___ | ___ | ___ | ___ | Scream or holler |
| ___ | ___ | ___ | ___ | Use foul language |
| ___ | ___ | ___ | ___ | Call names |
| ___ | ___ | ___ | ___ | Put partner down, say demeaning things |
| ___ | ___ | ___ | ___ | Criticize frequently or continually |
| ___ | ___ | ___ | ___ | Make fun of a disability or shortcoming |
| ___ | ___ | ___ | ___ | Make jokes at partner's expense |
| ___ | ___ | ___ | ___ | Ridicule or insult partner |
| ___ | ___ | ___ | ___ | Create fear with your voice |
| ___ | ___ | ___ | ___ | Yell in partner's face ("nose to nose") |
| ___ | ___ | ___ | ___ | Manipulate with lies and contradictions |
| ___ | ___ | ___ | ___ | Insult or drive away partner's family or friends |
| ___ | ___ | ___ | ___ | Ridicule or insult partner's religion, heritage, race, class, beliefs |

**EMOTIONAL ABUSE**

*Domination*

____ ____   ____ ____   Act like the boss
____ ____   ____ ____   Try to tell partner what **he/she can or can't do**
____ ____   ____ ____   Force partner to do things against his/her will
____ ____   ____ ____   Treat partner as less than your equal
____ ____   ____ ____   Make important decisions without consulting partner
____ ____   ____ ____   Refuse to do your share of chores

*Intimidation*

____ ____   ____ ____   Prevent or impede movement
____ ____   ____ ____   Use physical size to frighten
____ ____   ____ ____   Create fear with actions, gestures, and facial expressions
____ ____   ____ ____   Remind partner of ability to hurt him/her
____ ____   ____ ____   Drive recklessly to frighten
____ ____   ____ ____   Have weapons your partner is afraid of
____ ____   ____ ____   Threaten regularly to leave or to make partner leave the relationship
____ ____   ____ ____   **Threaten to hurt partner's family or friends**
____ ____   ____ ____   Threaten to take away children
____ ____   ____ ____   Threaten to hit, hurt, or abuse children
____ ____   ____ ____   Threaten to hit, hurt, or abuse partner
____ ____   ____ ____   Threaten to kill partner
____ ____   ____ ____   Threaten to hurt or kill yourself

*Humiliation*

____ ____   ____ ____   Ridicule or ignore feelings
____ ____   ____ ____   Ridicule or embarrass in public
____ ____   ____ ____   Ridicule or embarrass in private
____ ____   ____ ____   Force to do demeaning or degrading things
____ ____   ____ ____   Talk about an affair (real or invented) to hurt partner

*Harassment*

____ ____   ____ ____   Refuse to leave partner alone
____ ____   ____ ____   Follow around the house
____ ____   ____ ____   Stalk partner
____ ____   ____ ____   Accuse partner of being unfaithful

*Isolation*

____ ____   ____ ____   Prevent or discourage partner from seeing family or friends
____ ____   ____ ____   Refuse to let partner leave the house
____ ____   ____ ____   Refuse to let partner go to work or school
____ ____   ____ ____   Take away car keys or money
____ ____   ____ ____   Refuse to socialize with partner
____ ____   ____ ____   Refuse to let partner be alone in public
____ ____   ____ ____   Monitor partner, interrogate about where he/she has been

*Withdrawal*

____ ____   ____ ____   Withhold approval, appreciation, or affection to punish
____ ____   ____ ____   Withhold sex to punish
____ ____   ____ ____   Sulk angrily to get even

*Self-destruction*

____ ____   ____ ____   Hit or injure yourself
____ ____   ____ ____   Place yourself in dangerous situations
____ ____   ____ ____   Attempt suicide

_Using the children_
Turn children against partner
Use visitation to harass partner
Punish or deprive children when angry at partner

_Destruction of property and pets_
Threaten to destroy property
Drop plants or dishes
Break a window
Punch or kick a wall, door, doorjamb, etc.
Slam doors
Smash objects (TV, stereo, phone, remote control)
Destroy something of emotional significance
Threaten to harm a pet
Neglect, harm, or kill a pet

**SEXUAL ABUSE**
Express intense jealousy
Tell demeaning sexual jokes
Treat others as sex objects
Show sexual interest in others when with partner
Have an affair when you agreed to be monogamous
**Minimize importance of partner's feelings about sex**
Criticize sexual performance or frequency
Insist that partner dress more seductively or less seductively
Insist on unwanted touching or other sexual activity
**Threaten to retaliate if partner isn't interested** in sex
Force partner to watch pornography
Force your partner into sexual activity

**FINANCIAL ABUSE**
Completely control the finances
Refuse to let partner have his/her own checkbook
Make partner ask for money
Threaten to hurt partner financially
Take money or steal property
Threaten to withdraw financial support
Refuse to pay your share of bills as agreed

**LEGAL SYSTEM ABUSE**
Violate a restraining order
Violate a child custody agreement
Lie about partner to police or in court

*FIRST INCIDENT:*

*LAST INCIDENT:*

*WORST INCIDENT:*

Source: Shepard, M. F., & Campbell, J. A., *Journal of Interpersonal Violence* (Volume 7, Issue 3), Pages 291–305, copyright © 1992 by SAGE Publications, Reprinted by Permission of SAGE Publications

## Notes

1. Hawkley, L. C., Masi, C. M., Berry, J. D., & Cacioppo, J. T. (2006). Loneliness is a unique predictor of age-related differences in systolic blood pressure. *Psychology and Aging, 21*(1), 152; House, J. S., Landis, K. R., & Umberson, D. (1988). Social relationships and health. *Science, 241*(4865), 540; Kiecolt-Glaser, J. K., Malarkey, W. B., Chee, M., Newton, T., Cacioppo, J. T., Mao, H. Y., & Glaser, R. (1993). Negative behavior during marital conflict is associated with immunological down-regulation. *Psychosomatic Medicine, 55*(5), 395–409; Caspi, A., Harrington, H., Moffitt, T. E., Milne, B. J., & Poulton, R. (2006). Socially isolated children 20 years later: Risk of cardiovascular disease. *Archives of Pediatrics & Adolescent Medicine, 160*(8), 805–811; Thurston, R. C., & Kubzansky, L. D. (2009). Women, loneliness, and incident coronary heart disease. *Psychosomatic Medicine, 71*(8), 836; Hawkley, L. C., Masi, C. M., Berry, J. D., & Cacioppo, J. T. (2006). Loneliness is a unique predictor of age-related differences in systolic blood pressure. *Psychology and Aging, 21*(1), 152; Hawkley, L. C., Thisted, R. A., Masi, C. M., & Cacioppo, J. T. (2010). Loneliness predicts increased blood pressure: 5-year cross-lagged analyses in middle-aged and older adults. *Psychology and Aging, 25*(1), 132; among other studies.
2. Vaillant, G. E. (2008). Aging well: Surprising guideposts to a happier life from the landmark study of adult development. Tatkin, S. (2012). *Wired for love: How understanding your partner's brain and attachment style can help you defuse conflict and build a secure relationship.* New Harbinger Publications. (2008). *Hold me tight: Seven conversations for a lifetime of love*, p. 26. Little, Brown.
3. Coyne, J. C., Rohrbaugh, M. J., Shoham, V., Sonnega, J. S., Nicklas, J. M., & Cranford, J. A. (2001). Prognostic importance of marital quality for survival of congestive heart failure. *The American Journal of Cardiology, 88*(5), 526–529; Luo, Y., Hawkley, L. C., Waite, L. J., & Cacioppo, J. T. (2012). Loneliness, health, and mortality in old age: A national longitudinal study. *Social Science & Medicine, 74*(6), 907–914; Holt-Lunstad, J., Smith, T. B., & Layton, J. B. (2010). Social relationships and mortality risk: A meta-analytic review. *PLoS Medicine, 7*(7), e1000316; Patterson, A. C., & Veenstra, G. (2010). Loneliness and risk of mortality: A longitudinal investigation in Alameda County, California. *Social Science & Medicine, 71*(1), 181–186; Perissinotto, C. M., Cenzer, I. S., & Covinsky, K. E. (2012). Loneliness in older persons: A predictor of functional decline and death. *Archives of Internal Medicine, 172*(14), 1078–1084; among other studies.
4. Coan, J. A., Schaefer, H. S., & Davidson, R. J. (2006). Lending a hand social regulation of the neural response to threat. *Psychological Science, 17*(12), 1032–1039.
5. Hawkley, L. C., Masi, C. M., Berry, J. D., & Cacioppo, J. T. (2006). Loneliness is a unique predictor of age-related differences in systolic blood pressure. *Psychology and Aging, 21*(1), 152.
6. Coyne, J. C., Rohrbaugh, M. J., Shoham, V., Sonnega, J. S., Nicklas, J. M., & Cranford, J. A. (2001). Prognostic importance of marital quality for survival of congestive heart failure. *The American Journal of Cardiology, 88*(5), 526–529.
7. Kiecolt-Glaser, J. K., Newton, T., Cacioppo, J. T., MacCallum, R. C., Glaser, R., & Malarkey, W. B. (1996). Marital conflict and endocrine function: Are men really more physiologically affected than women? *Journal of Consulting and Clinical Psychology, 64*(2), 324.
8. Cohen, S. (2001). Social relationships and susceptibility to the common cold. *Emotion, Social Relationships, and Health*, 221–223, and Cohen, S., Doyle, W. J., Skoner, D. P., Rabin, B. S., & Gwaltney, J. M. (1997). Social ties and susceptibility to the common cold. *JAMA, 277*(24), 1940–1944.
9. Pekovic, V., Seff, L., & Rothman, M. (2007). Planning for and responding to special needs of elders in natural disasters. *Generations, 31*(4), 37–41, and Semenza,

J. C., Rubin, C. H., Falter, K. H., Selanikio, J. D., Flanders, W. D., Howe, H. L., & Wilhelm, J. L. (1996). Heat-related deaths during the July 1995 heat wave in Chicago. *New England Journal of Medicine, 335*(2), 84–90.

10. House, J. S. (2001). Social isolation kills, but how and why? *Psychosomatic Medicine, 63*(2), 273–274.

11. Feeney, B. C. (2007). The dependency paradox in close relationships: Accepting dependence promotes independence. *Journal of Personality and Social Psychology, 92*(2), 268.

12. Johnson, S. (2008). *Hold me tight: Seven conversations for a lifetime of love*. Little, Brown.

13. Bejerot, N. (1980). Addiction to pleasure: A biological and social-psychological theory of addiction. *NIDA Research Monograph, 30*, 246.

14. U.S. Department of Health and Human Services. (2009). *Results from the 2007 National Survey on Drug Use and Health: Detailed tables*. Substance Abuse and Mental Health Services Administration. SAMHSA, Office of Applied Studies.

15. Alexander, B. K., Beyerstein, B. L., Hadaway, P. F., & Coambs, R. B. (1981). Effect of early and later colony housing on oral ingestion of morphine in rats. *Pharmacology Biochemistry and Behavior, 15*(4), 571–576.

16. Tatkin, S. (2018). We do: Saying yes to a relationship of depth, true connection, and enduring love. *Sounds True*, 145–146.

17. Levine, A., & Heller, R. (2019). *Attached: Are you anxious, avoidant or secure? How the science of adult attachment can help you find – and keep – love* (Main Market ed.). Bluebird, p. 21.

18. Makinen, J. A., & Johnson, S. M. (2006). Resolving attachment injuries in couples using emotionally focused therapy: Steps toward forgiveness and reconciliation: Attachment theory and psychotherapy. *Journal of Consulting and Clinical Psychology, 74*(6), 1055–1064.

19. Levine, A., & Heller, R. (2019). *Attached: Are you anxious, avoidant or secure? How the science of adult attachment can help you find – and keep – love* (Main Market ed.). Bluebird.

20. Merrill, S. M. (2018). *An exploration of the transition from romantic infatuation to adult attachment*. ProQuest Dissertations Publishing.

# 4   What Is Prodependence?

Prodependence is a new psychological term the authors have created to offer an attachment-focused lens through which we can more effectively evaluate and treat loved ones of addicts.[1] The term itself, Prodependence, is a deliberate play on the word "Codependence," as that model (Codependence) has been so broadly identified as the sole method by which we have viewed this population. In many ways, the term Prodependence is a synonym for what attachment theorists describe as healthy interdependence *as applied to addiction treatment.*

Prodependence is specifically intended to offer a strength-based view of relationship dependency in those whose lives are being affected by a loved one's active addiction. This new model is offered because, as stated previously, the preexisting and ubiquitous Codependence paradigm is more focused on the deficits of intimate caregivers than on their inherent strengths. Codependency theory implies that such caregivers are responsible for enabling the addictive process by loving "too much," not in the right way, or related to internal trauma-based deficits. Prodependence approaches the matter differently, choosing to celebrate and take a healthful view of those who provide ongoing support to a beloved but deeply troubled other.

Using Prodependence as a guide, there is no shaming or blaming such people by telling them that the ways they've provided help are *wrong* or that they are *part of the problem.* With Prodependence, the desire to give of oneself to help rescue someone from addiction is never seen as pathology; thus, no one is ever "diagnosed" as Prodependent. Rather, the term is used to describe in positive interdependent terms *all efforts* given by a caregiver to maintain meaningful connection with a troubled loved one. Prodependence views the act of loving and trying to help an addict or a similarly troubled individual heal (or simply make it through the day), as an indicator of healthy love, healthy attachment, and unwavering interdependency in the face of extremely difficult circumstances.

In colloquial terms, acting in a Prodependent manner can be seen more as a compliment than a judgment because we, as therapists, are encouraged to normalize (rather than pathologize) the understandable actions taken when a loved one is failing. Prodependence provides recognition and validation for all efforts given when attempting to help a struggling loved one, along with hope and useful direction toward the caregiver's own healing. Using attachment

DOI: 10.4324/9781003058359-6

theory as a guide, Prodependence offers a prosocial lens of psychological health and a more nuanced view into the inner-world and lived experiences of the caregivers of troubled loved ones.

Consider the words of Dr. Stan Tatkin: "We learn to love ourselves precisely because we have experienced being loved by someone. We learn to take care of ourselves because somebody has taken care of us. Our self-worth and self-esteem also develop because of other people."[2]

Sadly, in modern Western culture, being dependent on others is generally viewed as a sign of weakness. We are taught from birth, regardless of our gender, that we are best served by going it alone and not asking others for help. Ultimately, we are told that our success and happiness are almost entirely dependent on our own strengths and abilities. We grow up learning that independence, self-sufficiency, and making it through life without deeply leaning into others for support is the right path and maybe the only road to self-actualization, even though an immense amount of research tells us the exact opposite is true.

Prodependence does not ever consider efforts made to help a loved one heal as pathology, even if those attempts to help are misdirected or ineffective. Under no circumstances does Prodependence imply that how we love can ever be viewed negatively. Instead, Prodependence acknowledges that loving an unpredictable, addicted partner who blames, lies, seduces, manipulates, and gaslights to keep using or behaviorally acting out can make pretty much anyone look and act a bit crazy.

When addicts become destabilized and unpredictable, when they start hurting themselves and others and their day-to-day functioning begins to falter, seemingly without resolution, those close to them are, by definition, in crisis. And people in the midst of such crises can look and act crazy. But that doesn't mean that they are. As with Codependence, Prodependence recognizes that when a caregiver's actions run off the rails, they can be redirected toward more effective solutions. However, Prodependence does not imply that a caregiver's dysfunctional behaviors arise out of any past or present trauma or pathology. Instead, Prodependence views their actions as an attempt to maintain or restore healthy attachment.

The expressions of pain and fear that we see with loved ones of active addicts are the same with Prodependence and Codependence. The primary difference lies in how we, as therapists, frame the problem to our clients and ourselves. One model is positive and supportive and meets a loving caregiver where they are; the other is the exact opposite, imposing a pseudo-pathology that often leaves such clients more self-doubting than self-assured.

While addressing similar concerns in the same population, these two models approach this work from vastly different perspectives. Codependence, as a deficit-based trauma model, views loved ones of addicts as traumatized, damaged, and needing help. Prodependence, as a strength-based attachment-driven model, views loved ones of addicts as heroes for continuing to love and remain attached despite the debilitating presence of addiction.

Prodependent treatment with caregiving loved ones of addicts recognizes and accepts, first and foremost, that these individuals are in crisis and likely to feel and behave accordingly. They may be emotionally labile, often exerting nearly super-human efforts to fill in the emotional and the practical deficits created by a troubled other. They may lose themselves in lists and chores, obsess about childcare and doctor's visits, look for bottles, research addiction, and compulsively manage ever-present financial concerns. They can lose sight of personal goals, gain (or lose) weight, and stop social and recreational activities to focus on their loved one's addiction. Internally, they experience rage, anxiety, fear, and depression, all of which can externally manifest as nagging, controlling, and hypervigilance.

From our perspective, caregiving loved ones' profound shift in focus from self to other represents nothing more than an anguished attempt to stabilize their lives (and families). Using the lens of Prodependence, we view such feelings and behaviors as more attributable to love and deep emotional commitment than as an expression of disease even though their actions and behaviors may not be useful or effective toward reducing or eliminating the addictive problem.

Prodependence validates caregiving in all forms as the loving act that it is. Prodependence views caregiving loved ones of addicts not as innately damaged, but as relatively healthy people responding to an abnormal situation (addiction in a loved one) as best they can. Do loved ones of addicts always make the best decisions and go about the business of helping in the best possible way? Of course not. Do they occasionally overstep their bounds in ways that are harmful to themselves and the people they are trying to help? Yes, they do. Do they at times nag, cajole, rage, beg, blame, pull, push, withdraw, and all the rest? Of course. But why would we expect anything different from a person in the midst of a profound crisis?

The simple truth is that loved ones of active addicts are perpetually in crisis. Naturally, they try to overcontrol the addict to solve the painful problems. In the process, they can panic and make bad decisions. They may overdo. They may help ineffectively. They may inadvertently enable and appear to be pathologically enmeshed. But that does not mean they are psychologically disordered. What it means is they are *people in crisis*, behaving in the ways that people in crisis tend to behave. After all, how many family members of addicts learned in elementary or high school how to effectively manage such situations? Not many. Prodependence says that they are simply doing their loving best – no more, no less.

Our job as therapists, when such individuals come to us for help, is not to pathologize them. Instead, we need to validate their experience, value their contributions, and guide them toward the development and implementation of useful and effective solutions.

Prodependence says:

> You're a wonderful, strong individual for putting so much effort into helping your struggling loved one. I am so impressed with all the work you have done to stay by their side. It's possible, however, that you're not helping them as effectively as you'd like. But who can blame you for that? It's hard to worry about loving someone in the best possible way when you're living in the middle of a disaster zone. If the house is burning down, you

grab your loved one and you drag that person out of the fire, and you don't worry about whether you're grabbing too hard, or in a way that hurts. But now that you are in counseling and no longer alone with all of this, we can help you figure out how you might help your struggling loved one more productively – in ways that might be more useful to your relationship and that leave you feeling better supported and less overwhelmed.

Prodependence encourages us to celebrate humankind's natural and healthy need to develop and maintain intimate attachments and to provide ongoing, uninterrupted support to loved ones – even in the face of addiction or some other profoundly troubling life crisis. Moreover, Prodependence moves the locus of "the problem" away from the often-overwhelmed caregiver and family members, while validating their feelings of love and hope (and anger, fear, sadness, exhaustion, etc.).

When working with the Prodependence model, we work to reframe any misguided attempts to help their loved one out of addiction and into health. No matter how ineffective, even harmful a caregiver's behaviors may have become, we acknowledge them for their efforts.

In this way, Prodependence seeks to validate, empathize, and actively help these clients in the here and now, rather than encouraging them to step back, self-reflect, and take a deep dive into "their own issues."

## As Addiction Is Stigmatized, So Are Caregivers

Despite everything we now know about addiction – what causes it, why some people are more psychologically or biologically susceptible than others, and how to treat it – addiction is viewed in nearly every culture (and in most families) as shameful, and silence is encouraged. Because of this, spouses, parents, siblings, and others who care for addicted loved ones tend to suffer in silence, providing care as best they can but with little or no useful guidance. There's too little information; there's too much shame; there's what the neighbors will say; etc.

Families of addicts desperately work to "look good" on the outside while they collapse internally. And when the problem is finally brought to light, the advice they often receive is to intervene (pushing the addict toward treatment) and then to detach and distance themselves from the problem. And woe to those who choose otherwise, as they will surely be blamed, shamed, and pathologized as enmeshed, controlling, and contributing to the problem. In short, they will be labeled as Codependent, meaning they are psychologically troubled, just like the addict, and their primary path forward is uncovering their unresolved trauma and related behaviors so they can fix whatever it is they've been doing wrong.

How is this helpful? Why pin the stigma of addiction on the addict's nonaddicted, well-meaning loved ones as well as (and sometimes more than) on the addict? Why would we negatively label hard-working, deeply loving, intensely loyal, profoundly afraid, nearly exhausted loved ones of active addicts as

Codependent or worse? Is this the kindest and most effective way to invite them into the healing process? Does this represent the empathetic, nonjudgmental embrace that such people clearly need and deserve? We think not.

No wonder it's tough to keep loved ones of addicts involved in treatment. These are individuals who've spent months or even years trying to keep their lives and families intact, with little if any thanks for their efforts, and now they've got a therapist who is talking to them (or maybe at them) in ways that cause them to feel blamed, shamed, and at fault.

Frankly, we find it hard to understand why any counselor or therapist would initiate a therapeutic relationship with a client who is already painfully overwhelmed and under-supported by defining their empathic caregiving as pathology. And when such clients fail to embrace or even rebel against this concept, we call them difficult, thereby reinforcing the inaccurate and harmful belief that they are as innately troubled as the addicts they love. Otherwise compassionate professionals who view such clients through this type of deficit-based lens can be heard to complain about these "difficult and troubled" patients, saying things like:

- They don't want to own up to their part in the problem.
- They view the addict as the sole source of the problem, and that makes it hard to help them.
- They don't see how their attempts to be caretakers are making things worse.
- They may be sober, but they're every bit as sick as the addict and sometimes sicker.
- They just can't stop rescuing, and that causes more problems than it solves.

## Being an Addict and Loving an Addict Are Different Clinical Problems

What if loved ones of addicts aren't really so difficult? What if the source of their supposedly difficult nature is an external crisis (the addiction) rather than some internal pathology? What if the problem with loved ones of addicts lies more in how we conceptualize them than in the caregivers themselves? What if our primary model for treating them has misunderstood and marginalized them in ways that simultaneously confuse them and cause them to feel unnecessarily blamed and shamed? What if we, as therapists, automatically pathologize loved ones of addicts as Codependent and therefore driving a dysfunctional family system? What happens when our Codependent "diagnosis" pushes them into a reactionary state where they feel more defensive in our work than supported? What if our current models leave them spinning around in circles while we play pin the tail on the pathology?

Prodependence advises that such de facto, predetermined, and pejorative views of any client are not reflective of effective, empathetic therapy or counseling. As caregivers ourselves, we can be kinder and more effective by leading with curiosity, empathy, compassion, and support, rather than judgment.

Even when caregiving loved ones have been "doing it all wrong," experience has taught us that it's usually not a good idea to tell them that or to blame them in any way for facilitating and perpetuating someone else's dysfunction. And why would we expect otherwise? If you were the loved one of an addict and you were exhausting yourself by working part-time in three different places while taking care of multiple people in ever more challenging situations, would you feel engaged by a message that asks you to look at *your problem*? Most likely you would not, because this message would feel both hurtful and counterintuitive.

If our therapeutic approach to loved ones of addicts alienates them before they can take advantage of the care and insight that we can offer, then perhaps the time has come to change our methodology. The authors seek a more empathetic and compassionate way to approach caregiving loved ones of addicts. And then, instead of criticizing them for resisting a path that feels innately wrong to them, we can approach them with a less critical, less shaming model.

## Prodependence Is Attachment-Based and Crisis-Focused

To treat loved ones of addicts using Prodependence, provided they are not exhibiting meaningful signs of mental health disorders or addictions themselves, we need not find that anything is "wrong with them." We can simply acknowledge the trauma and inherent dysfunction – the crisis – that occurs when living in close relationship with an addict, and then we can address that in the healthiest, least shaming way.

Interestingly, Prodependence generally recommends and encourages many of the same therapeutic outcomes as Codependence, most notably a fresh or renewed focus on self-care coupled with implementation of healthier boundaries. That said, the models approach this work from vastly different perspectives. Codependence, as a deficit-based trauma model, views loved ones of addicts as traumatized, damaged, and needing help. Prodependence, as a strength-based, attachment-driven model, views loved ones of addicts as heroes for continuing to love and continuing to remain attached despite the debilitating presence of addiction. Heroes in crisis, but heroes nonetheless.

In short, the Prodependence model encourages therapists and clients to celebrate a client's natural and healthy human need to develop and maintain intimate connections, and to provide ongoing, uninterrupted support to loved ones – even in the face of addiction or some other profoundly troubling life crisis.

The expressions of pain and fear that we see with loved ones of addicts are the same with Codependence and Prodependence. Again, the primary difference here lies in *how we frame the problem* to our clients and ourselves. One perspective allows us to support our clients by meeting them exactly where they are – that is, in crisis – while the other is the exact opposite, imposing a pseudo-pathology that often leads to unnecessary shame and remorse.

Once the crisis stage of healing is passed, if a client wants to do deeper forms of inner work (like addressing unresolved trauma), that's great. And that often is what occurs. When the dust has finally settled and the addiction is being adequately addressed, clients who have the interest, the resources, and the time might say, "I'm beginning to wonder if anything about the way I grew up might relate to my having chosen this person or to my having tolerated all of their dysfunction?" At that point, the door is open for deeper work. However, in the early stages of treatment, that's just not where the client is likely to be. And attempting this deeper psychodynamic work too soon typically leads a client not to crisis resolution, better boundaries, and improved self-care, but to increased anxiety, self-doubt, and a sense that they are part of the problem.

This type of shame is counterproductive. Rather than labeling and pathologizing loved ones of addicts for defending and refusing to distance themselves from their caregiving roles, our job as therapists is to thank them for their efforts and encourage them to continue their pursuit of love and emotional intimacy, though in healthier, more Prodependent ways.

## Clinicians Appear to Prefer Prodependence

After initially formulating his thoughts and ideas about Prodependence and the model's advantages over the older yet problematic Codependence model, Dr. Rob Weiss formulated a study[3] to assess whether addiction therapists, 83% of whom said they work with both addicts and loved ones of addicts, after a brief education about the Prodependence approach, felt like Prodependence is a better model for working with loved ones of addicts and similarly troubled individuals. This study focused on the clinical treatment of spouses and partners of behavioral addicts, but it seems reasonable to extend the findings to not only other addictions and similarly troubling issues. After all, the desire for healthy attachment is the same no matter the crisis.

To test the concept of Prodependence and its appeal to addiction treatment specialists, Dr. Weiss created a 30-question survey, with 18 questions asked first, followed by a one-hour educational presentation about the concept and proposed methodology of Prodependence, followed by 12 more questions. In particular, Dr. Weiss wanted to understand how these therapists viewed the clinical needs of this client population before learning about Prodependence vs. after learning about Prodependence. After viewing the presentation, objective measures showed a measurable, profound, and meaningful shift in the responses of those therapists surveyed. When participating professionals, most of whom had practiced some version of the Codependency model for years or even decades, were offered a more attachment-focused, crisis-aware, and non-exploratory method of evaluation and treatment – that is, Prodependence – they strongly preferred the newer approach.

In this research, Dr. Weiss found that even though 89.4% of participating therapists believe that spouses and other loved ones of addicts are likely to be in crisis in their first 60 days of treatment, the vast majority (81.8%) will nonetheless default to evaluation and treatment planning methods sourced in early-life trauma (such as Codependency) and/or couples' relationship functioning, rather than aligning their initial approach toward attachment and crisis-focused treatment models.[4]

Moreover, the majority (62.55%) indicated that they were somewhat likely to very likely to suggest early in treatment that loved ones of addicts learn about Codependency – and furthermore, this would be their plan even before having met or seen said clients.[5]

Please consider this point for just a moment. Where else in our therapeutic world would we *ever* diagnose a client before meeting them online or in-person? Even when reading evaluations of a given person before we meet them, we are taught to leave our assumptions at the door when the client enters. So, a de facto assumption that if a client is in a relationship with an addict, the client must *automatically* be traumatized, enmeshed, and controlling (i.e., Codependent) does not align with the basic ethical tenets of our profession.

This may be why the clinicians in this study almost uniformly expressed concerns about the Codependency model, with many of those concerns centering around the fact that there is no one model of Codependency or Codependency treatment. To this point, a strong majority (79.69%) of participants stated that they felt they'd had to "wing it" to some extent when working with loved ones of addicts, despite Codependency being the current treatment standard.[6] More importantly, when presented with the attachment-focused, crisis-aware basics of Prodependence, participants almost uniformly expressed strong preference for the new approach. Weiss writes:

> After viewing the presentation, there was a measurable, profound, and meaningful shift in the responses of those therapists and professionals surveyed. Based on the simple information above, it becomes clear that when professionals are brought back to the basics of the codependency model as written by its progenitors and then are offered newer, more crisis-oriented, strength-based, relational, and non-exploratory methods of evaluation and treatment, that respondents preferred newer evaluation and treatment methods/models over those they had previously endorsed *less than one hour prior.*[7]

The subjective response to the Prodependence paradigm was also uniformly positive. Participants made statements such as:

- I believe [Prodependence] will be effective because it offers support and guidance without inadvertently shaming or blaming the loved one.
- [Prodependence] is a more positive and useful way to approach partners.
- I love the term.... Great way of staying positive, showing support, and letting [clients] know you care.
- I believe [Prodependence] more accurately and effectively treats the needs of loved ones and spouses.[8]

Nearly all the data provided, both objective and subjective, showed that a random sample of addiction-focused clinicians, without exposure to a new model such as Prodependence, will choose assessment and treatment paradigms more out of prior education, habit, (decades-old) training, and deeply held personal beliefs than by accurately following validated treatment methods already proven to be most effective in crisis-driven cases. Utilizing clinical techniques focused on introspection and self-exploration when working with clients in the midst of a life crisis is by definition counterproductive to achieving early client rapport and actively helping them in the early stages of treatment. In spite of this fact, the model of Codependency and related early-trauma exploration are so deeply ingrained among self-identified experts in addiction treatment that these models have essentially become the de facto paradigm, regardless of client need, regardless of the fact that it's been decades since the introduction of Codependency and there is still no universally validated diagnosis or even a universal understanding about what defines Codependency, much less the best way to treat it (should it exist at all).

Sadly (for our clients and their families), educational efforts toward attachment-focused crisis models like Prodependence have essentially been overruled by Codependency. It appears that powerful word and related forms of evaluation and treatment have become so deeply ingrained in the culture of the addiction treatment world as to have drowned out and superseded paradigms that have been advanced in mental health care, especially those defined by modern attachment theory. Thus, the need for this book.

## Notes

1. Weiss, R. (2018). *Prodependence: Moving beyond Codependency*. Health Communications, Inc.
2. Tatkin, S. (2012). *Wired for love: How understanding your partner's brain and attachment style can help you defuse conflict and build a secure relationship*. New Harbinger Publications.
3. Weiss, R. (2019). Prodependence vs. codependency: Would a new model (Prodependence) for treating loved ones of sex addicts be more effective than the model we've got (codependency)? *Sexual Addiction & Compulsivity, 26*(3–4), 177–190.
4. Weiss, R. (2019). Prodependence vs. codependency: Would a new model (Prodependence) for treating loved ones of sex addicts be more effective than the model we've got (codependency)? *Sexual Addiction & Compulsivity, 26*(3–4), 177–190.
5. Weiss, R. (2019). Prodependence vs. codependency: Would a new model (Prodependence) for treating loved ones of sex addicts be more effective than the model we've got (codependency)? *Sexual Addiction & Compulsivity, 26*(3–4), 177–190.
6. Weiss, R. (2019). Prodependence vs. codependency: Would a new model (Prodependence) for treating loved ones of sex addicts be more effective than the model we've got (codependency)? *Sexual Addiction & Compulsivity, 26*(3–4), 177–190.
7. Weiss, R. (2019). Prodependence vs. codependency: Would a new model (Prodependence) for treating loved ones of sex addicts be more effective than the model we've got (codependency)? *Sexual Addiction & Compulsivity, 26*(3–4), 177–190.
8. Weiss, R. (2019). Prodependence vs. codependency: Would a new model (Prodependence) for treating loved ones of sex addicts be more effective than the model we've got (codependency)? *Sexual Addiction & Compulsivity, 26*(3–4), 177–190.

# Section 3

# Conceptualizing Prodependence Treatment

# 5 The Underpinnings of Prodependence Treatment

## What Is Prodependence?

Prodependence can be thought of as a synonym for interdependence. Both terms imply that within any relational system (a family, for example), there is a complementary balance of individual strengths and vulnerabilities that evolve over time to help maintain consistency and stability. This balance is in a constant state of flux based on internal and external stressors to the system or family.

Prodependence views the impact of addiction on the family as one such threat to the stability of primary interdependent relationships. In such cases, the needs and vulnerabilities of the struggling individual will most often overwhelm the coping skills of the other(s), thus pushing the system into crisis. The Prodependence model encourages a return to homeostasis by – in part – supportively steering caregiving loved ones back toward healthy coping. As they become more resilient with the strength-based support and direction of Prodependence, balance can be restored.

Prodependence applies current attachment theory and research to a population that has long been considered "codependent." This new model encourages clinicians to reevaluate how we assess and provide treatment to such people by viewing them as victims of circumstances beyond their control and not as inherently broken people. The goal of this approach is to move beyond labeling and pathologizing such individuals by viewing them and their behaviors through a strength-based, non-pathological lens.

In short, Prodependence views loved ones of addicts as having been destabilized by the crisis of addiction. Thus, the model *does not* focus on "trauma repetition" or "over-enmeshment" (i.e., Codependency). The Prodependent belief is that people in the midst of a profound life crisis don't need analysis or self-examination. What they do need is active support, direction, and hope.

Prodependence recognizes that loved ones of active addicts are in crisis simply because a meaningful attachment relationship is being threatened by an active, progressive disease (addiction). To put this colloquially, who among us

DOI: 10.4324/9781003058359-8

would not become fearful, hypervigilant, out-of-control, and/or regress to less functional ways of coping when attempting to navigate this type of situation?

## Treating the Crisis at Hand

By shifting our clinical focus away from the exploration of early trauma and intra-psychic dysfunction, Prodependence allows us to more fully work in the here and now. This new paradigm encourages treating clinicians to directly validate, support, and direct clients toward coping with the immediate crisis, rather than exploring whatever issues this acute problem may or may not have evoked within them. Crisis intervention and emotional stabilization are now our primary clinical tasks.

The following are the two themes addressed by Prodependence when working with this caregiving population that will invariably shift based on client need.

1.  The *current external crisis* that arises out of living in an out-of-control situation. The work here involves therapists being clinically active by providing support, direction, and education to reduce client anxiety, confusion, and shame. We must work to help such clients negotiate the difficult landscape of their "here and now" problems.
2.  The *active internal crisis* that occurs because the client is facing the failure and potential loss of a deeply meaningful interdependent relationship. In other words, we work to normalize and validate all of the client's feelings and behaviors by framing them as being typical of anyone facing similar losses and fears. No judgment, no analysis.

Working within a crisis model requires counselors to lean into the client's strengths, rather than emphasizing the client's vulnerabilities. Crisis intervention treatment helps to improve client functioning by focusing on issues such as restoring hope, stabilization, grounding, normalizing, resourcing, etc. – all while allowing us to align with the client's immediate concerns.

The introduction of Prodependence reflects a new characterization and view of people facing meaningful and out-of-control attachment losses due to addiction. When we view such clients as exhibiting nothing more than a normative response to their current circumstances, our work becomes clear and present. We are not working with broken people. We are simply working with people who are struggling to cope and are *feeling broken* by their very painful present.

## Defining Crisis

Crisis is a state of emotional turmoil or an acute emotional reaction to a powerful stimulus or demand. There are five distinct elements commonly present someone experiencing an interpersonal crisis, such as when a loved one is addicted.

1. *Emotional*: The usual balance between thinking and emotions is disturbed. There will be clear evidence of psychological, emotional, physical, or behavioral impairment, or a combination of these with the struggling loved one.
2. *Coping*: Previously successful coping mechanisms have failed.
3. *Regression*: Individuals experiencing a traumatic interpersonal crisis often partially revert or regress into past states or behaviors due to the stressful nature of their situation. For example, someone with a past history of compulsive eating may revert back to that behavior when dealing with the loss of an aging parent.
4. *Impairment*: Evidence of impairment in an individual or family. Within the relational system, there is an apparent circumstance or situation that is causing the destabilization and crisis within the given system.
5. *Remorse*: People experiencing a profound loss – and there are many profound losses with addiction – are going to feel remorse. Remorse is a part of grief. It is not uncommon for individuals in a crisis to repeatedly blame themselves for whatever they think they might have done differently to help. Remorse in such situations may sound something like this: "If only I had done this or that, maybe I could have prevented the addiction or kept it from getting to this point. Why didn't I pay more attention? Was I not doing my part?"

## The Brain in Crisis

One way to view mental health is to see it as a balance between emotional reactivity and intellectual insight. Too much emotional activity is a problem, as the client will be unable to be objective about their circumstances. Too much intellectualization can also be unproductive as it may lead to denial and escalation of the problem. When in crisis, the usual balance between thinking and feeling is disturbed. This is automatic and unconscious. Part of our work with clients in crisis is to assess where this balance lies within an individual client, which provides us with the information needed to best help both in the moment and over time.

The following is an image depicting the specific parts of the brain that are activated when a traumatic experience occurs (crisis). The "automatic" responses that an individual typically experiences while in crisis include fighting back (fight), running away (flight), and shutting down (freeze). When a client is in a fight/flight/freeze state, that person is completely overwhelmed. To prevent or recover from such responses, individuals need help making sense of their circumstances by shifting their internal experience of the current trauma from the limbic system (the "feeling" part of the brain) to the executive system (the "thinking" part of the brain).

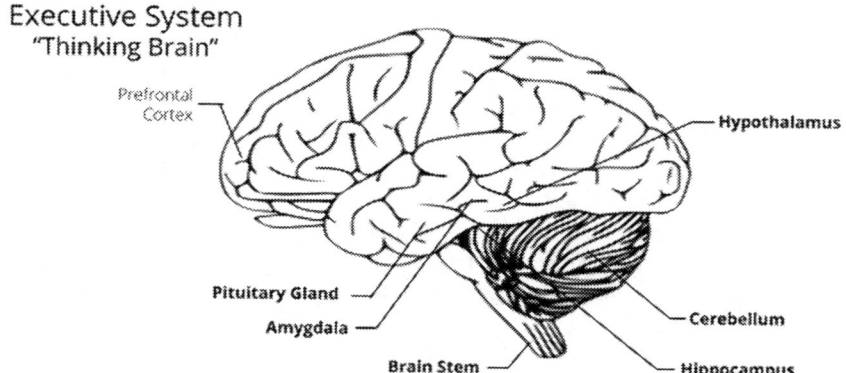

Executive System
"Thinking Brain"

Prefrontal Cortex

Hypothalamus

Pituitary Gland

Amygdala

Cerebellum

Brain Stem

Hippocampus

**Limbic System**
**"Feeling Brain"**
*Trauma response, emotion, and addiction live here.*

The executive or intellectual parts of the brain are primarily located in the prefrontal cortex. That is where higher thinking and reasoning occur. If a fearful or painful trauma occurs, more primitive parts of our brain take over, shutting out the prefrontal cortex. This is a functional evolutionary development meant to help keep humans alive in immediate crisis situations. For example: If I see my young child racing across the street in front of a truck I don't think, I act. In that moment, my heart races, my thinking is singularly focused on that situation, and thus I lose access to intellectual thought as my adrenaline-fueled response kicks in. Such masking neurochemicals allow me to execute the actions required to meet this emergency without hesitating or falling apart.

This automatic, unconscious response to trauma has evolved over thousands of years, and it is why complex problem solving, analyzing, and regulation is difficult for loved ones of addicts when they're in the earliest stages of treatment – that is, still in crisis. As such, they have less access to intellectual thought and tend to be far more emotionally reactive than they were prior to the crisis. This is a reminder of why *therapists should never attempt to diagnose someone who is in the midst of a crisis*. We simply have no idea about the individual's normative level of functioning. Clinicians working from a crisis perspective understand the need to pay careful attention to limbic activation in clients, exercising patience with self-discovery and self-actualization until the client stabilizes and becomes less reactive, thereby more able to reengage the prefrontal, or executive part of their brain.

*Example*:

The 45-year-old wife of an active alcoholic comes to therapy feeling "unstable, overwhelmed, numb, and frightened." The source of her panic was the discovery that her husband had not only been drinking during the day, but leaving work to get drunk with sex workers throughout their 17-year marriage. As she sits in the therapist's office for the first time, attempting to explain what has happened, she becomes confused, agitated, and begins to sob uncontrollably.

After several attempts to compose herself, she eventually explains to the therapist that she is having trouble remembering the details about all that is happening and that everything seems to be running together. She describes how she is feeling dizzy and nauseous and would feel better if she could lay her head down for a few minutes. The therapist, recognizing that the client is having a trauma (limbic brain) response simply by discussing her current circumstances, immediately stops questioning her and moves to help regulate and normalize her physical and emotional symptoms. This therapist understands that assessment questions can wait until the trauma reactivity has passed. In such moments, the locus of treatment moves from content to process in order to help the client self-regulate and gain stability.

## The Foundational Beliefs of a Prodependent Therapist

Prodependence is an interpersonal attachment and strength-based model that sees a caregiving loved one's commitment to helping an addicted family member as both heroic and reasonable given the gravity of the injuries (and other crises) they've experienced in the relationship.

Prodependence is based on the following principles:

- Human beings are internally wired for secure attachment and pair bonding (interdependence).
- Disruptions in such attachments can create a primal pain response.
- A primal pain response initiates a sense of crisis.
- An active crisis state stops the individual from accessing their intellectual self.
- Individuals in this state will often engage in frantic (and sometimes misguided) attempts to stop and/or control the crisis that is the source of their emotional instability.
- An addict's choice to abuse substances or act out behaviorally should *never* be ascribed to the faults of the family, partner, or caretaker. Addicts use because they choose to use. Period.
- It is abusive to put responsibility on anyone other than the addict for the addict's decision to use or behaviorally act out.
- Loved ones of addicts are deeply affected by the addict's instability on an almost daily basis.

- Loved ones of addicts experience painful losses and circumstances due to the addiction.
- The desire to help or save an addicted loved one should *never* be viewed as pathological.
- No pathology should ever be attributed to someone's attempts in trying to rescue, save, or control a loved one who is out of control.
- No one can be addicted to another person.
- It is not possible to "love too much."
- Trying to save a troubled loved one is hero's work that should be validated and normalized.
- No caregiver can offer perfectly aligned support. Some of what caregivers do may be effective and some will not, but it is unacceptable to blame them for not having given in "the right way" or the most productive way.
- Crisis intervention techniques and modalities are best utilized in such situations to help loved ones regain as much emotional and intellectual equilibrium as possible, often while in the midst of navigating painful, unstable circumstances.
- The therapist's goal is to stabilize, normalize, educate, and help such clients find their way forward. Nothing more, nothing less.

## Viewing the Models Side by Side

It may be useful here for the reader to view a few differences in the language and intent of Codependence treatment vs. Prodependence treatment. Next you will find a list of clinical themes most often addressed when working with loved ones of addicts. The goal here is to note the meaningful differences between the two models in terms of language and clinical stance. To gain insight into these differences, we will continue to utilize the case of the previously mentioned overwhelmed wife of an alcoholic.

### Clinical Theme: Trauma Repetition

- *Codependence Therapist*: "I wonder if the abandonment and betrayal you experienced with your father may have caused you to choose a partner who would also betray and abandon you in adult life (your alcoholic husband). Maybe some of those unmet childhood needs have left you willing to put up with just about anything to keep your husband close to you – no matter how much it hurts you. It may well be true that if you hadn't been raised by such a troubled dad, then you wouldn't have chosen this relationship in the first place. As you heal your past, you will make better relationship decisions in the present. You may even find, over time, that this wasn't ever the right relationship for you."
- *Prodependence Therapist*: "I can see that you have been doing everything in your power to help your addicted husband, only to come up short. What a nightmare this is for you, because no matter how much you love and

want to make it work with him, his behaviors are out of your control. No wonder you feel so crazy. No wonder you hurt so much. No wonder you are exhausting yourself trying to make things better. Of course, feelings from the past are going to come up in a situation like this. But for now, let's just focus on the current crisis. If you'd like to explore some of your history once all of this has passed, we can follow that path later."

### Clinical Theme: Remaining Close to the Addict in Order to Help

- *Codependence Therapist*: "Sadly, it feels like you are following the same patterns in this adult relationship that you had in your childhood with your father. Your obsessive and understandable fear of being abandoned by this man has led you to stay around and tolerate his drinking. Ultimately, you are neglecting yourself while trying to help him. I wonder what it would be like if you could stop worrying so much about him and instead refocus on you."

- *Prodependence Therapist*: "One of the clear strengths I see in you is the ability to do whatever you can to hang in there with someone you deeply love, despite the pain it may cause you. Even though some of your actions have not resulted in his getting sober, I admire your commitment to doing everything you can to make your family whole. I can see that you are a lot stronger than you feel yourself to be. Now that you have my help, perhaps together we can work to tackle the nightmare you find yourself in today."

### Clinical Theme: Doing Whatever It Takes to Help Solve the Problem

- *Codependence Therapist*: "Since chaos and being left behind are such common threads throughout your life, perhaps you are working a lot harder than you should to make this right. I wonder if all this anxiety and your attempts to rescue your spouse are more about trying to resolve your own past losses in this hauntingly familiar situation. When you do this, you feed your own denial about how little power you really have over all this. I think you will see this more clearly as you learn how your past is affecting your present."

- *Prodependence Therapist*: "If I were in your shoes, I would do whatever I could to make this better, too. I have no doubt that what's going on today is a reminder of what you went through in the past. That must make it harder for you. Nonetheless, your past pain is not the reason you continue to love and help your husband with hope in your heart. You are doing all this out of love, not past losses. In fact, there isn't anything wrong with what you are doing; you just need more help doing it. Let's put the past aside for the moment so we can find some practical ways to help make all this better. Later on, when your life is more stable, we can address those past issues if you choose to do so."

### Clinical Theme: Relationship Addiction

- *Codependence Therapist*: "Children who feel unloved and unwanted, like you did when you were young, often develop an addiction to the 'need' to be loved. We find that people who choose to be in addicted relationships often find that they themselves become addicted – to the addict, as well as the desire to rescue the addict from the addict's own chaos. Because these kinds of addictive patterns may be less obvious, your addiction to him – your Codependence – may be difficult to see. Let's take a look at the ways that, like any addict, you use denial to avoid seeing *your part* in the problem."

- *Prodependence Therapist*: "I know why you stayed with him. You love him. You still see the best in him, even when he is hurting you and himself. In many ways, I think you are holding out for the good moments you have shared in this relationship, hoping they will return. I want to help you to stay hopeful and to stop blaming yourself for not being able to resolve this problem. It didn't start with you. The person you love is troubled and all addicts have their own internal struggles. He would have found himself in the same situation no matter what you may or may not have done."

### Clinical Theme: Rescuing the Addict

- *Codependence Therapist*: "It feels like you are more hurt than helped by doing so much for the addict. As you work on your own problems, you will gain insight into the ways your love for your addicted husband pushes you into your own form of denial. Once that happens, you will be able to differentiate between loving blindly vs. seeing him for who he really is. He needs to fix this problem on his own without your help. You need to step back and let him struggle on his own. Otherwise, your enmeshment with him is going to continue to make things worse."

- *Prodependence Therapist*: "There is nothing wrong with you for doing everything in your power to try to make this better. Despite the painful loss of trust that his addiction has caused, you still love him. Naturally, you want to make him better. After all, we are wired to bond and do our best to help, save, and rescue those we love from pain."

### Clinical Theme: Detachment, Setting Boundaries, and Distancing from the Addict

- *Codependence Therapist*: "An important way to stop addictively focusing on your partner is to focus more on yourself and on your own healing. This is best done by detaching with love. In other words, you need to love the addict from a distance so you will not get sucked back into his drama so easily. As part of therapy, we need to find ways to remove you from this mess so you can work on yourself while the addict finds other sources of support."

- *Prodependence Therapist*: "Of course you want to help your husband heal and work through his struggles. I'm here to help with that. But let's be clear, there's nothing wrong with your desire to stay connected to him despite the fact that he is making such a mess of his life and yours. You are doing and feeling what all of us do and feel when we love someone who is deeply troubled. You are trying to help. Given that, I think our work here is more about setting boundaries to help you learn where your assistance is effective and where it is not. We both want your loving support to be more productive, but this does not mean stepping aside or away from him. Today, he likely needs you more than ever, whether he can see that or not."

## A Note about Codependence

The authors of this work fully understand the opportunities a life crisis can create for long term personal growth. However, as we have repeatedly stated, someone in an acute relational crisis is unable to focus on such higher goals. This doesn't mean that we discount the effectiveness of this work or the growth that it can offer us; we simply believe that when caregivers and loved ones of addicts are facing active addiction or early recovery in a loved one, *this is not the time to delve into their past.*

Further, the fields of psychotherapy and addiction treatment had already created readily understandable, research-sourced concepts to describe problematic dependencies, terms and diagnoses which were unfortunately washed away and subsumed by the Codependency movement. As terms like unhealthy dependency, overdependency, enmeshment, trauma repetition, and Dependent Personality Disorder were valid, almost universally understood terms prior to the introduction of Codependence, the authors believe there is not now nor was there ever a place in formal diagnoses or treatment planning for the concept of Codependence.

It is our sincere hope that mental health and addiction providers will reclaim such previously acknowledged terms when providing longer-term, insight-oriented forms of therapy. In this way, we suggest that the terms Codependence and Codependency be confined to colloquial/pop-culture use and no longer utilized to define client presentation, diagnosis, or treatment method.

## Stages of Codependency Treatment

In the 1980s, Timmen Cermak suggested four treatment stages for recovery from Codependency.[1] We will discuss that model here (though there are countless other approaches) because Dr. Cermak's work is both foundational and typical of Codependency work in general (meaning other approaches are generally variations of Cermak's).

Cermak's first and second stage treatment goals (outlined next) are in direct contradiction to what we now know to be effective in early treatment for loved ones of addicts and other individuals experiencing interpersonal crises.

### *Codependence Treatment*

Stage 1: Treatment for the Reidentification Stage

- Treatment Goals

  ○   Help clients to begin dismantling their denial system.
  ○   Help clients to focus attention back on themselves.
  ○   Help clients to begin recognizing how they are perpetuating their own problems.

- Treatment Approach

  ○   Continually comment on the existence of the clients' denial.
  ○   Form empathic connections with the clients, otherwise they will have no tolerance for your comments about their denial.
  ○   Assume the clients are in pain, as this will make the empathic connection easier to create.

Stage 2: Treatment for the Survival Stage

- Treatment Goals

  ○   Help clients to solidify their identity as Codependents.
  ○   Help clients to work through the grieving process that accompanies the loss of the illusion of power.
  ○   Bring clients to a new awareness of compulsivity.
  ○   Initiate an investigation into the realistic limits and uses of willpower.

- Treatment Approach

  ○   Assertiveness training, communication skills, and giving information about the multiple symptoms seen in Codependence.
  ○   Reinterpret the past and present.
  ○   Explore how they went about controlling their feelings, avoiding personal needs, and how they tried to "make" others love them to feel better about themselves.
  ○   Reframe the clients' inability to abstain from compulsions as a measure of their unwillingness to feel.[2]

Stages 3 and 4 focus on problematic Codependent behaviors. However, the treatment for these would extend beyond the initial crisis. We will not examine these stages in detail here as they are contraindicated when working within a crisis. That said, in Stage 3, Cermak focuses on core issues such as how Codependency has infiltrated all areas of life – further exacerbated by attempts to control the addict. In Stage 4, Cermak focuses on the client's Codependency-free reintegration into a normal life, including termination of the therapeutic relationship.

Cermak's model is a clear example of the pervasive beliefs and thought processes held by Codependence-based clinicians regarding loved ones of addicts.

## Stages of Prodependence Treatment

Prodependence takes a five-stage approach focused primarily on helping clients restore healthy coping. The primary initial treatment goal of this model is to guide clients toward a return to their prior level of functioning – essentially who they were before their world fell apart.

The Prodependence approach recognizes that individuals in crisis are ill-equipped in the early stages of treatment for in-depth personal work. Thus, the model proposes that therapists' primary focus in the early stages of treatment should be on skill-building, resourcing support, educating, and creating emotional stabilization and not intrapsychic investigation.

The expectation of the Prodependent therapist is not for the clients to achieve self-actualization through long-term interventions and therapy; instead, the expectation is that the clients will develop the ability to better self-regulate and have useful helping and coping strategies available when needed. This, of course, aligns with the most effective general crisis intervention treatment approaches.

### Prodependence Treatment

The five stages of Prodependence treatment are as follows:

1. *Normalization and Mitigation of Crisis*: When individuals seeking therapeutic help are in a relationship crisis, they want, more than anything, to feel better. They want their life to go back to normal. They want to resume the normal thoughts, feelings, and activities available to them before their lives spun out of control. They want answers to questions like "Does everyone in my situation experience this?" and "Can people really heal from this?" They want to know that they are not crazy and that what they are experiencing is human. What they do not want is to talk about their "role" in the problem or how their current situation may be reminiscent of (even a reenactment of) past trauma.

2. *Support and Connection*: A prevailing need for individuals experiencing relational difficulties is to know that they are not the only ones who are going through or have been through the type of trauma they are experiencing. They often carry high levels of shame and find themselves taking responsibility for the behavior of their loved one. They also tend to be isolated in their pain and unsure of who to confide in. Challenging their shame and offering reassurance that their situation is not an isolated one is a key component of treating the crisis.

3. *Basic Information and Education*: Providing clear and concise information and education about the clients' experience will help the clients manage the extreme fear and hopelessness that may accompany it. Helping the clients visualize a path forward without overburdening them with all the particulars is a tricky balance that falls on the treating therapist. The information

provided must be hopeful but also realistic. Future projections about positive outcomes for the relationship should be avoided; however, reassuring the clients about their ability to navigate and find the best solutions throughout the healing process will generate confidence and reassurance.

4.   *Offering Hope*: The therapist must strike a careful balance between providing some hope while simultaneously managing expectations of future outcomes, particularly with the struggling loved one's healing process. Offering a realistic path for the caretaker's journey also requires the clinician to be mindful of the unique personal details of that person's life, avoiding overgeneralizations about him or her or the situation.

5.   *Giving an Overview of Healing*: Creating a generalized overview of the healing path ahead for both the clients and the clients' addicted loved one helps the clients plan ahead and manage their expectations as bumps in the journey naturally and inevitably arise. In addition, this overview can help the clients in their future decision-making process.

These five stages will be explored in further detail in Chapter 6.

## Treatment Outcomes

The hope with *Codependence-oriented treatment* is that the clients, after resolving (or not resolving) the immediate crisis, will achieve a higher level of functioning than before the crisis struck. This involves taking them on a journey of self-discovery, with the ultimate goal being client self-actualization and improvement.

The challenge here is it requires the patient, while in the midst of an acute trauma, to be introspective and analytical about themselves and their experiences, this despite the fact that when trauma responses are keeping clients in "survival mode," higher reasoning and executive functioning are unavailable to them. As such, the most likely outcome of Codependence treatment is that after resolving (or not resolving) the immediate crisis, the clients feel blamed and shamed for a problem not of their own making. And with that, they either leave treatment or regress to a lower level of functioning.

Prodependence approaches treatment differently, starting with its view of caregiving loved ones of addicts as individuals who are, first and foremost in crisis, and in need of crisis-focused treatment. Because of this, identifying trauma, self-actualization, and self-improvement is removed from the early-stage treatment equation. The focus instead shifts to normalization, support, education, hope, and healing. The client then feels welcomed, understood, and supported.

With this type of therapeutic alliance, the work of healing a damaged relationship – letting go of the "need" to control another person's behavior, learning to help in more productive (and welcomed) ways, and engaging in better self-care – is far more likely to occur.

The shorter – and longer-term results of the Prodependence approach, therefore, are that the client, after resolving (as best they can) the immediate crisis, returns to some degree of normalcy in their life. Personal coping skills are developed and implemented to reduce stress and other crisis symptoms. At the same time, less intrusive and therefore more effective helping skills are developed and implemented. Down the line after the client and the client's presenting crisis are sufficiently stabilized, if the client chooses to do deeper, more introspective work, that work can take place *without the client feeling blamed or shame or pathologized.*

We believe the Prodependent approach is far more likely to achieve lasting positive results because it recognizes:

- Loved ones of addicts are in crisis, and it is abusive to confront or "pathologize" someone in an active crisis.
- There is plenty of trauma to deal with in the here and now when loving an active addict. A heavy focus on historical trauma may result in missing the client's immediate needs.
- Loved ones of addicts are not acting out an addiction. Loving and caring for an addict, even an active addict, is not an addiction.
- Clients in crisis require supportive, crisis-aware treatment, rather than judgment and blame.
- It is never a clinician's job to force self-actualization on anyone. If patients work through their initial crisis in a healthy way and then want to engage in self-actualization at a later date, that's great. But forcing self-actualization and self-reflection while someone is in the middle of a crisis is counterproductive.
- While the ideal resolution of a crisis brings personal growth and insight to our clients, this is not required for healing, as most clients we see simply want things to get better.

## Language to Avoid, Language to Embrace

Prodependence is more than just a new approach to treatment. It offers a 180-degree turn away from the kinds of Codependency-focused language that can feel highly judgmental and devaluing to clients.

Language matters. Words matter. Our clients are listening. The use of words or phrases such as "obsessed," "controlling," "manipulative," "enmeshed," "in denial," "unstable," etc., should be avoided. This terminology, even when well-intended and accurate, applies a shameful, pathological-sounding label on behavior and feelings that are typical of any person in an acute crisis. By utilizing such terms, we are likely to exacerbate the individual's preexisting feelings of fear, shame, and self-doubt, rather than normalizing and validating their experience.

As the focus of a Prodependence-based therapist is on the client's strengths and real-time experiences, the language we utilize is neutral. By employing words and phrases such as "worried," "concerned," "trying to help," and "attempting to feel safe," we validate the client's understandable desire to protect a deeply important relationship. Even in situations in which the client's efforts to help are leading to a negative result, the source of those desires is viewed as arising out of love rather than pathology. Thus, the language used to discuss, diagnose, and help loved ones of addicts must reflect this more positive view.

Consider the following graph, which compares Codependency language to Prodependence language.

| Codependent Language | Prodependent Language |
|---|---|
| Enmeshed | Deeply involved |
| Externally focused | Concerned about the welfare of others |
| Enabling | Supporting |
| Fearful | Concerned |
| Lacking healthy boundaries | Eager to care for a loved one |
| Can't say no | Chooses to say yes |
| Obsessed with the addict | Determined to protect the addict and family |
| Living in denial | Unwilling to give up on a loved one |
| Angry | Fearful of further loss with no control |
| Controlling | Trying to be heard |
| Hypervigilant | Anticipating problems |

Although the Codependence and Prodependence models have several similar goals (e.g., boundary-setting, self-care, meeting needs, etc.), they do not share language in terms of how therapists think about or speak to the client. One of the primary differences between the models is in the way the therapist clinically defines, frames, and approaches the problem the client is experiencing.[3]

A Codependency-based therapist sees and refers to the client's functioning as impaired or disturbed resulting from early-life traumatic experiences, which the current situation provokes and exacerbates. A Prodependence-based therapist sees the very same client as a courageous individual who has most likely done all they can to help and save someone they love, to no avail. Is past trauma activated when any of us are in stressful, frightening situations like this? Sure, that's natural. But why would any professional point out or explore this so early-on as per Codependence, especially as these symptoms are most likely to diminish once the crisis has passed?

Looking through a Prodependent lens, the ways in which this client has attempted to help a struggling loved one may or may not be as useful or helpful as the client may have hoped. This does not deter us from viewing their motivation as driven by anything but a desperate desire to remain connected and safe, as opposed to being controlling and manipulative in response to their own early-life family dysfunction.

## Transference

### Client Transference

The phrase "Never question a positive transference" is particularly valid when working with families of addicts. From a Prodependent perspective, our job is for clients to view us as active helpers, not explorers of their internal uncharted territory. Should negative transference occur we strongly encourage an immediate and non-analytic return to connection. Prodependence doesn't ask us to examine transference but rather to lean into it when it is positive and quickly defuse it when it is not.

### Therapist Countertransference

Love is hard to find and even harder to maintain. Even the most trained among us are not immune to the pain, confusion, and losses that addiction and other illnesses bring when played out among our own children, families, parents, and spouses. Many of us can directly relate to our client's experiences in one arena or the other. And that can be a good thing. Unrelated to addiction, nearly everyone of us can relate to the painful impotence felt when someone we deeply love is deeply hurting but we cannot fix it, no matter how much we love them.

But all the empathy and compassion in the world doesn't help our clients get better if those feelings are more of a response to our own experiences than those of our clients. When we emotionally resonate with our clients' powerful stories, experiences, and emotions, they can lead us to play out our own issues with the client (our countertransference). Being tempted to "take on our clients' battles," related to our own internal responses and life experiences, defines the term countertransference. Thus, the better trained among us attend our own therapy if only for this reason. Being better armed with insight into our own reactivity and history makes us less likely to act them out in real time with our clients.

## Notes

1. Cermak, T. L. (1986). *Johnson Institute Books professional series. Diagnosing and treating co-dependence: A guide for professionals who work with chemical dependents, their spouses and children.* Johnson Institute Books.
2. Cermak, T. L. (1986). *Johnson Institute Books professional series. Diagnosing and treating co-dependence: A guide for professionals who work with chemical dependents, their spouses and children.* Johnson Institute Books.
3. Weiss, R. (2018). *Prodependence: Moving beyond Codependency.* Health Communications, Inc.

# 6 Foundations of Clinical Practice

## Keep It Simple

When commencing treatment, the primary role of the Prodependent therapist is to facilitate initial client interactions that are simple and straightforward while simultaneously acknowledging and addressing their immediate circumstances. Support and feedback should be readily understood, and any direction provided must be clear, concise, and applicable near fully focused on the here and now. Most importantly, the therapist must create an environment of validation, hope, and reassurance. One of our primary objectives is to not "tip the scale" on an already overwhelmed system.

- *Simplicity*: In a crisis, people respond best to simple procedures. Simple things have the best chance of having a positive effect.

  - *Therapist*: "Since you are struggling to sleep at night, let's try a simple relaxation exercise (or app) that you can use as you prepare to go to bed. Let's also talk about what to do if you can't sleep. I find it is often best to simply get out of bed for a bit to watch TV rather than tossing and turning in the dark."

- *Brevity*: Psychological first aid needs to be short and precise.

  - *Therapist*: "You seem understandably upset today about all that has happened. Let's talk less today and relax more. I would like you to close your eyes and take a few deep breaths. Then we'll do a quick somatic (body) check in to see if you can recognize when and how your stress affects you physically."

- *Concrete Direction and Support*: Use creativity. Specific instructions may not exist for every case or circumstance.

  - *Therapist*: "Let's talk about dinner tonight. You said that eating has been hard for you, that you are often not hungry. This is understandable, as you are in crisis and people in crisis sometimes don't feel like eating. If it's OK with you, I think it might be useful to plan a menu for tonight and tomorrow night's dinners – healthy foods that

DOI: 10.4324/9781003058359-9

you typically enjoy eating. After you eat tonight, you can leave me a brief voicemail to let me know how it went. And don't forget about dessert!'"

- *Pragmatism and Validation*: Keep it practical. Impractical suggestions can cause the person to feel more frustrated and out of control. Encourage healthy functioning.

  ○ *Therapist*: "The tension in your body is obvious. That makes sense, as you are carrying so much weight on your shoulders. Let's pick out a place where you can get a massage, or let's find a stretching or yoga class. Working out some of your physical stress is likely to make everything just a bit easier."

- *Work in the Here and Now*: Clients in crisis do not have the psychological sophistication to engage in in-depth clinical evaluations or discussions of the past. Remain focused on the problems at hand.

  ○ *Therapist*: "I understand why all of this reminds you of what happened with your mom when she got sick and you were little. The situation now likely feels out of control just like it did when you were little. I hear you, and I get it. Old wounds often arise when we are in a crisis. But for now, we need to get you feeling stronger and less stressed. That means that this may not be the best time to delve into the past, as it might overwhelm you further. Now let's get back to talking about what to do tonight if your sister comes home high …."

- *Offer Hope*: Set up reasonable expectations of a positive outcome. Encourage the individual in crisis to recognize that help is present, there is hope, and the situation is manageable.

  ○ *Therapist*: "I don't know if your relationship will survive all it has gone through, but I do know that the love you have shared will always live inside of you. We have to take this day-by-day for now. I will hold onto hope for you, though: hope that your relationship will heal and hope that, if relationship healing is not your path, you will at last find peace and meaning out of all this pain and loss."

## The Five Stages of (Crisis-Oriented) Prodependence Treatment

As stated in Chapter 5, there are five stages of crisis treatment. Those stages, because partners and other loved ones of addicts are, by definition, in crisis when they enter treatment, transfer directly to the Prodependence model. As a reminder, those five stages are:

1. Normalization and Mitigation of Crisis.
2. Support and Connection.

3.   Basic Information and Education.
4.   Hope.
5.   Healing.

### Stage 1: Normalization and Mitigation of Crisis

According to Richard James and Burl Gilliland,

> A crisis occurs when a person is confronted with a critical incident or stressful event that is perceived as overwhelming despite the use of traditional problem-solving and coping strategies. Often, it is not the event itself that causes the crisis; rather, it is the appraisal of the event as serious, uncontrollable, and beyond the patient's resources for coping that triggers a crisis response.[1]

This phenomenon is never more evident than when loved ones who are dealing with out-of-control relational losses seek out our assistance. They have either been living with or have just been exposed to a situation that feels well beyond their ability to remedy.

When implementing a crisis treatment intervention, the first steps are to help normalize what the clients are experiencing and to assist in lessening the immediate negative impact of the situation where possible. When clients are literally living with an addict's bad decisions –which are imploding their most important relationships, the natural effect is an explosion of internal confusion and pain. Most clients in this situation look to the therapist to provide reassurance that they are not alone and that others have experienced similar things and lived through them. They want to know that they are a "healthy" person caught up in a crisis they didn't cause and are not capable of fixing on their own. They need to know that anyone in this kind of situation is going to feel the way they feel and act the way they act. They need to know that there are other people going through this same thing who can offer hope and support because they are there or have been there. They need to know that we can help.

*   *Client*: "I can't believe my son actually stole money from me to buy drugs. Why can't he just be a normal kid like my sister's son, who is a straight A student?"
*   *Therapist*: "If you look on Facebook or talk to friends, it can feel like everyone else's child (and family life) are functioning much better than yours, but we both know that that is not true. There are many parents, kids, and families going through the exact same issues as you. In fact, I am going to show you some of the places where you can connect to such people."

Whether or not the therapist agrees with the client's assessment of the situation is not relevant at this stage. Clients don't need (or want) factual clarification in this emotional arena. What they need is to feel understood, supported, and validated for everything they feel. Assuring the clients that what they are experiencing matters and is typical given their situation is the order of the day.

## Stage 2: Support and Connection

People in relationships with active addicts are living amid disrupted attachment. As the addict pulls away from them to focus on the relationship with an addictive substance or behavior, this can leave caregivers and other loved ones feeling alone, betrayed, and rejected. Worse still, the potentially shameful nature of the issues will often keep such people from reaching out to their typical sources of support. This is where Prodependent therapists come in.

Healers since time immemorial have innately understood that one of the most effective ways to validate and move people beyond profound life difficulties is to encourage their active involvement in a supportive community. Long before we had therapists, we had community.

In modern times, we can seek communities specific to our issue via online support groups, group therapy, or a 12-step program, along with safe and empathetic family, friends, and loved ones. Keep in mind that the first thing we do with an isolated, mentally ill person is to bring them into connections with us and others. The first thing we do to help an addict heal is to bring them into a cohort of community (AA and the like). Why would we not do the same for loved ones of these troubled people? A supportive community allows for healthy interdependent attachments to occur with others are in a similar situation. Thus, we help ease the burden of loneliness and isolation that loved ones of addicts so commonly experience.

Examples of supportive communities:

- Support groups for loved ones of addicts – moderated or unmoderated.
- Clinical therapeutic groups.
- Safe and empathetic family and friends.
- Church/religious community.
- Online groups.
- Workshops and other forms of care that are supportive and safe.

Often, therapists want their clients to take responsibility for finding their own support groups. This is especially important when treating addicts, as they need to learn how to be accountable for their own process of healing. This is not, however, the best approach with caregivers and other loved ones of addicts. In these cases, our job is different, and we must take a more active role in resourcing and evaluating where our client might find and receive the most useful support. Thus, we should:

- Encourage them to find trustworthy individuals with whom they can share their story.
- Educate them on how to use boundaries for safety when sharing their story.
- Encourage them to participate in a psychotherapy, 12-step, or other support group when available and appropriate.

- Assist them in identifying safe individuals and places to turn to in an emergency.
- Provide information and resources.

The ability to engage healing support from a community of others will in great part determine the long-term outcomes for both the addict and the addict's loved ones. It is understandable that some people, especially those who are not themselves addicted, might wrestle with this concept. That said, loved ones of addicts often feel alone, confused about the proper course of action, and unsure of who to talk to about what they are experiencing and feeling. Many keep their confusion and fears bottled up because they worry that they might be judged for the bad decisions and behaviors of their addicted loved one. In short, they are uncertain of how to find trustworthy and empathic support when they are suffering and alone. They are ashamed and afraid.

So, again, stable support should come from people who encourage self-care and compassion, not those who give advice or add to pain and confusion. It is not helpful if someone in the client's support network tries to fix the client or offers unsolicited opinions, no matter how well-intended. Helpful healing support holds space for feelings and experiences while encouraging (but not dictating) a plan for healthy living.

- *Therapist*: "I know this idea may seem uncomfortable, even like the last thing you want to do right now, but this is a time when I really need you to trust my experience. We need to help you to find and join a safe, consistent support group, or at least discuss how you can identify a network of trustworthy individuals. You need people outside of therapy for you to confide in, get support from, and connect with, as this is one of the fastest ways to get you back on your feet and feeling like your old self again."
- *Client*: "You know I really prefer to keep these issues to myself. I'm not really a group kind of person. And let's face it, I'm not the one who needs a group to get well. I'm not the one who is addicted and hurting my family. Plus, I don't want to hang out with a bunch of other hopeless, depressed, and overwhelmed people."
- *Therapist*: "It is understandable that you would feel uneasy about sharing your story with others, as it is so personal and it is difficult for you to trust right now. However, since the connection with your addicted loved one has been injured, it will help for you to get some connection and support from others who won't judge you or give you advice. Right now you really need people who can just listen and be unconditionally supportive. And I really want you to find some useful role modeling and guidance from people who have been exactly where you are but are a few steps further down the road than you."

### Stage 3: Basic Information and Psycho-Education

When working with clients who are in an acute relational crisis, the therapist should consistently provide basic instruction and learning throughout the

nitial phase of treatment. A steady flow of information and direction, offered
at a tolerable pace for each client, will help them stabilize and gain insight.
This offers them a more stable foundation from which they can make the difficult relational decisions that they will most likely face in the future. Keep in
mind that most people don't understand the addictive process, the meaning of
crisis, or the gut-wrenching feelings of interpersonal betrayal and grief. Thus,
the information and psycho-education provided should focus in areas such as:

- Addiction.
- Attachment.
- Crisis and trauma.
- Relational betrayal.
- Grief and loss.
- Self-care.
- Seeking support.
- Personal needs.
- Abuse.
- Boundaries.
- Grounding and stabilization.
- Healing and repair.

This is where therapists need to take an active role in terms of recommendations for videos, books, podcasts, articles, and other sources of readily digestible
information. Recovering from a crisis does not mean a sole focus on feelings.
All of us, every day, live in the worlds of our social relationships, emotions *and
our intellect*. To ignore one in favor of the other is to do our clients a disservice.

To this end, therapists should keep updated lists of resources that can be easily given to and used by the client. Keep in mind that our tech-oriented world
offers endless guides toward information and healing. Be sure to use all the
video and audio resources available to aid this population. A book is great. But
when treating the overwhelmed client, finding content that they can watch or
hear is more likely to be effective.

### Stage 4: Hope

An ongoing task of a Prodependence-based therapist is offering the client
hope throughout the counseling process. While our active presence in their
lives may, in and of itself, provide a natural space for repair to commence,
we still need to say the words and say them often. We need to tell them that
theirs is not an impossible situation. We need to tell them that others have
healed through this and so will they. We need to tell them that recovering
from addiction happens every day in those who are willing to work at it. We
need to tell them that it is very possible to help restore themselves and their
loved one to health.

The clients' ability to be vulnerable and participatory in their own healing is
unquestionably more effective when we validate their (often heroic) attempts

to help their addicted loved one – even when those attempts may at times have been counterproductive.

Because the caregiving loved ones' world as they knew it has been shattered, it is often difficult for them to hold onto any sense of optimism and security. By the time they come to us, they are already feeling overwhelmed and hopeless. Hope is not a promise and it is not a solution, but by holding it for them until they can hold it themselves (and telling them so), we offer a lifeline to the struggling individual. Hope helps them to better tolerate their current anxieties and fears and can provide them with a vision for better days ahead. Hope is a powerful notion, one that we can use over and over again to support those we are tasked to serve. Be sure to use it often.

### Stage 5: Healing

In addition to understanding the basics of addiction, caregiving loved ones should be informed about what the path of personal and interpersonal healing may look like for them. To this end, therapists will need to address grief, interpersonal trauma, and self-compassion.

### Grief

A universal emotional challenge for loved ones of addicts is loss and grief related to the addiction. As therapists, our ability to predict this, recognize the impact, and speak to the grief the clients are experiencing is essential. In this way, we can help the clients gain insight and tolerance for their own lived experience.

In one small example, a client may say,

> Yes, my brother is using again, but why does that leave me in this horrible emotional place? What is going on with me that I feel so angry? I'm not even his wife or one of his kids, so why do I feel like somebody just died? I'm not doing well and feeling guilty even though I did nothing to cause this problem. Will these feelings ever end? Can I fix them myself or will I feel this way until he gets better, if he gets better?

Clients may also wonder if life will ever hold the meaning it once did, and what their purpose will be after all that has happened. Understanding grief can be viewed as a useful therapeutic tool used to help our clients create a different paradigm of their relationship or outlook on life.

As Viktor Frankl, a holocaust survivor and psychiatrist, stated, "When we are no longer able to change a situation, we are challenged to change ourselves..., to choose [our] attitude in any given set of circumstances, to choose [our] own way."[2]

As part of experiencing grief, it's important to ask clients to identify (even write a list) of their current and past losses. These losses, both large and small, can be connected to any area of life. For example, simply having your kid called out by a teacher for not doing their homework can feel overwhelming to someone who is already overwhelmed. Identifying, explaining, and normalizing the nature of their grief and loss improves resiliency and helps to reduce self-doubt.

### Interpersonal Trauma

The Prodependence model rests on the belief that we are healthier when we have ongoing, meaningful, supportive, mutually dependent relationships. So, as Prodependent therapists, we should strive to encourage and validate interdependence as a strength.

Addiction, however, creates profoundly disturbing rifts in previously stable relationships. Most such rifts are a form of interpersonal trauma. When important others lie to us, break our trust, ask us to believe their lies, and abuse our goodwill in order to drink, use, or act out behaviorally, interpersonal trauma is present.

Here are a few examples of relational values and beliefs – broken by active addiction – that lead directly to interpersonal trauma:

- Trust.
- Connection.
- Communication.
- Time.
- Safety.
- Friendship.
- Spirituality.
- Love.
- Companionship.
- Money.
- Sex.
- Hope.
- Stability.

As these losses accumulate, the ability to process and grieve them appropriately may not always be available. If so, the consequences can be profound. Some of the possible consequences of not grieving can include:

- Chronic health problems.
- Career disruptions.
- Memory problems.
- Relational challenges/changes.
- Too much or too little sleep.
- Compulsivity (cleaning, shopping, spending, etc.).
- Anxiety and depression.
- Social and/or emotional isolation.

- Poor self-care.
- Flare-ups of previously stable mental health concerns.
- Addiction or addiction relapse.
- Loneliness.
- Loss of trust in other current relationships.
- Lack of trust when exploring future relationships.
- Externalized or displaced feelings (most often anger).
- Spiritual pain and confusion.
- Role loss.

### Self-Compassion

A primary skill that will assist loved ones of addicts in the healing process is self-compassion. Self-compassion can adjust thought processes and behaviors toward the self to those in which clients can act as their own loving advocate and friend in times of pain. As Kristin Neff explains,

> Painful feelings are, by their very nature, temporary. They will weaken over time as long as we don't prolong or amplify them through resistance or avoidance. The only way to eventually free ourselves from debilitating pain, therefore, is to be with it as it is. The only way out is through.[3]

Individuals in interpersonal crisis may be accustomed to taking care of and worrying about a struggling loved one to the point of feeling exhausted, ashamed and empty. And why not, when they expend such a large percentage of their emotional and physical energy attempting to take care of the addict and to keep their relationship intact?

Some clients may have previously learned how to use affirmations to help change negative thought patterns and beliefs. Without question, building self-esteem and challenging unhealthy thinking through the use of affirmations is helpful, but fully engaging in self-compassion requires a bit more.

The active practice of self-compassion goes beyond convincing oneself that one is worthy and good enough with the use of repetitive positive thoughts. It speaks to the parts of self that are feeling pain and works to nurture and validate the imperfect self. It is rooted in the ability to be supportive and gentle with oneself in moments of pain and distress. It points out that pain is a part of our shared experience and a natural part of the human experience. Therefore, clients learning how to kindly support themselves through pain naturally brings increased feelings of self-worth and hope.

- *Example of an Affirmation*: "Even though I have been really hurt by my spouse, I am a good person who is worthy of love."
- *Example of a Self-Compassion Statement*: "It really hurts that my spouse has lied and deceived me, but I know that I'm not the only one who has felt

this way. It's OK to take whatever time I need to grieve so much of what has been lost."

Although employing tools and support are crucial to overcoming the crises we see with addiction, clients taking time to be gentle with themselves is also important. This will involve connecting with pain and distress by acknowledging it and supporting themselves through it. With clients in crisis, self-compassion can aid in both long-term healing and developing an internal sense of stabilization and self-efficacy. It can help rebuild the their inner world and ability to move forward, despite pain and uncertainty.

## Summary

Prodependence is a crisis-oriented approach to treatment for caregivers and other loved ones of active addicts. As such, the stages of Prodependence work mirror the stages of crisis work in general, with a step-by-step focus on:

1. Normalization and Mitigation of Crisis.
2. Support and Connection.
3. Basic Information and Education.
4. Hope.
5. Healing.

In the initial stages of Prodependence treatment, there is no focus on internal analysis or self-growth. More importantly, the clients are never blamed for the bad choices and behaviors of a person they choose to love. Nor are they shamed for continuing to love and care for that person. Instead, the Prodependent therapist meets such clients where they are – amid profound crisis – and proceeds accordingly.

In the following chapter, the specifics of such work are discussed in detail.

## APPENDIX

## Crisis Response Inventory (CRI)

Date
Client Name

This inventory is designed for individuals who have experienced crisis in their most intimate relationships, including partners and loved ones of addicts and similarly struggling people. The following inventory contains items from the PC-PTSD-5 screen designed to identify the impact of these symptoms. Read through each symptom and score the severity on a 1 to 5 scale, with 1 being mild and 5 being severe.

1.  Have you ever experienced nightmares about your loved one's behaviors?
    1 2 3 4 5

2.  Are you currently experiencing nightmares about your loved one's behaviors? 1 2 3 4 5

3.  Have you ever experienced unwanted thoughts about your loved one's behavior? 1 2 3 4 5

4.  At this moment, are you currently experiencing thoughts about your loved one's behavior? 1 2 3 4 5

5.  Have you ever tried to dismiss thoughts about your loved one's behavior?
    1 2 3 4 5

6.  Are you experiencing difficulty not thinking about your loved one's behavior right now? 1 2 3 4 5

7.  Have you ever avoided situations that remind you about your loved one's behavior? 1 2 3 4 5

8.  At the current time, are you experiencing the temptation to avoid situations that remind you of your loved one's behavior? 1 2 3 4 5

9.  Have you ever felt on-guard or watchful? 1 2 3 4 5

10. Are you experiencing feelings of being on-guard or watchful right now?
    1 2 3 4 5

11. Have you ever been easily startled? 1 2 3 4 5

12. At this moment, are you feeling easily startled? 1 2 3 4 5

13. Have you ever been numb or detached from people, activities, or surroundings? 1 2 3 4 5

14. At this moment, are you experiencing being numb or detached from people, activities, or surroundings? 1 2 3 4 5

15. Have you ever felt guilty or to blame for your loved one's behavior and/or the problems it has created? 1 2 3 4 5

16. At this moment, are you experiencing feelings of guilt or blaming yourself for your loved one's behavior and the problems it has created? 1 2 3 4 5

17. Have you ever felt intense fear, panic, or anxiety? 1 2 3 4 5

18. Are you experiencing intense fear, panic, or anxiety right now? 1 2 3 4 5

19. Have you ever felt out of control? 1 2 3 4 5

20. At this moment, are you experiencing a feeling of being out of control?
    1 2 3 4 5

21. Have you ever had outbursts of intense anger or rage? 1 2 3 4 5

22. Are you experiencing outbursts of intense anger or rage right now? 1 2 3 4 5

23. Have you ever experienced deep sadness or depression? 1 2 3 4 5

24. Are you experiencing deep sadness or depression right now? 1 2 3 4 5

25. Have you ever experienced hypervigilance or felt preoccupied with preventing your loved one's behavior from happening again? 1 2 3 4 5

26. At this moment, are you experiencing hypervigilance or feeling preoccupied with preventing your loved one's behavior from happening again?
    1 2 3 4 5

27. Have you ever experienced emotional irritability? 1 2 3 4 5

28. Are you experiencing emotional irritability at this moment? 1 2 3 4 5

29. Have you ever experienced an uncontrollable "flood" of emotions that washes over you? 1 2 3 4 5
30. At this moment, are you experiencing an uncontrollable "flood" of emotions that is washing over you? 1 2 3 4 5
31. Have you ever been constantly worried? 1 2 3 4 5
32. Are you experiencing constant worry right now? 1 2 3 4 5
33. Have you ever had constant thoughts about your loved one's behavior? 1 2 3 4 5
34. At this moment, are you experiencing continual thoughts about your loved one's behavior? 1 2 3 4 5
35. Have you ever had intrusive thoughts about your loved one's behavior that unexpectedly pop into your mind? 1 2 3 4 5
36. Are you experiencing intrusive thoughts of your loved one's behavior that have unexpectedly popped into your mind at this moment? 1 2 3 4 5
37. Have you ever had difficulty concentrating or remembering? 1 2 3 4 5
38. At this moment, are you experiencing difficulty concentrating or remembering? 1 2 3 4 5
39. Have you ever felt a sense of helplessness? 1 2 3 4 5
40. Are you experiencing a sense of helplessness right now? 1 2 3 4 5
41. Have you ever had sleep difficulties? 1 2 3 4 5
42. Are you currently experiencing sleep difficulties? 1 2 3 4 5
43. Have you ever experienced an increase in isolation in your nonprimary relationships? 1 2 3 4 5
44. Are you currently experiencing an increase in isolation in your nonprimary relationships? 1 2 3 4 5
45. Have you ever participated in excessive behaviors (e.g., eating, cleaning, working, exercise, alcohol, drugs, social media/blogging, shopping, religion)? 1 2 3 4 5
46. Are you currently participating in excessive behaviors (e.g., eating, cleaning, working, exercise, alcohol, drugs, social media/blogging, shopping, religion)? 1 2 3 4 5
47. Have you ever found yourself "policing" your loved one's behavior? 1 2 3 4 5
48. Are you currently feeling the desire to "police" your loved one's behavior? 1 2 3 4 5

TOTAL SCORE (odd numbers life span): _____
TOTAL SCORE (even numbers current): _____
TOTAL SCORE (odd plus even): _____
For therapist use only.

- Mild        48–72
- Low         74–120
- Moderate    122–168
- High        170–214
- Severe      216–240

## Notes

1. James R. & Gilliland B. (2012). *Crisis intervention strategies*. Nelson Education.
2. Frankl, V. E. L. (1992). *Man's search for meaning: An introduction to logotherapy* (4th ed.). Beacon Press.
3. Neff, K. (2011). *Self-compassion: The proven power of being kind to yourself.* William Morrow.

# 7 Clinical Applications of Prodependence

As we have emphasized throughout this text, when working with loved ones of active or newly recovering addicts, therapists should focus from day one on the immediate crises their clients are facing. In so doing, we build a more effective alliance and work ahead moves faster. There are no models to introduce, no books needed to explain *the clients' problems*. All we need to do is educate them about the nature of their understandable grief and the addiction-driven pain, loss, and hopelessness they're experiencing. This is how we build the kind of therapeutic alliance that allows the clients to view us as both empathic and engaged.

What we must push back against is the adoption of *any therapeutic framework* that encourages these already traumatized individuals to take a deep dive into their past traumatic dependency losses or early-life injuries. By working in the moment (rather than in the past) from the very start, we reduce and perhaps eliminate any need the clients may have to defend their prior actions. They simply feel supported for all they have done. Next is one of the best examples we can offer for why we reject Codependency and seek a more strength-based model.

## Jack and Yvette's Story

Jack comes to you for therapy because he cannot get his alcoholic wife Yvette to stop drinking. She is out of control, and he just can't handle it anymore. And so, he is in your office.

Yvette's alcoholism has led to her losing several jobs and being stopped for a DUI more than one time. The most disturbing thing to Jack is the fact that on many occasions (previously unknown to him), his wife has driven both their kids and some friends' children home from school drunk. Jack learned about this from a concerned neighbor and was immediately humiliated (and also terrified) by it.

Jack tells you what he's been doing to try to make the situation less dangerous for Yvette, their kids, and others. He also tells you that his ideas worked for a while but now are failing. He tells you that he tried every trick in the book to get Yvette sober or at least reduce her drinking. He says tearfully,

> I've cried, I begged, and talked to her about our children's future, all of which brought promises to never do it again. But then those promises are

DOI: 10.4324/9781003058359-10

broken. She won't go to treatment and she refuses to confront her problem. And we really needed her income and her help with the kids just to help us get by.

Then Jack tells you why he feels so ashamed.

About two years ago, after Yvette had lost yet another job, we made a bargain. I put an ice-cold bottle of vodka on the dining room table that day after dinner and said, "As long as you can keep your day job, do not drink and drive at any time – especially with our kids in the car – I will have a cold bottle of vodka ready for you here at home at 4:30 every night. You can drink as much as you want and I won't say a word, as long as you are done with work and the kids are home safe. But you have to stay home when you drink, and you can't drink during the day before 4:30."

Then Jack tells you that this plan actually worked. For a while.

For the next 18 months, I had a wife who held onto a job, brought our kids home safely, and didn't get in trouble with the law. Better yet – more often than not – she was able to stay sober until after dinner. For me, this was a big win. It gave me the ability to do my job, to be a good father, and to protect our family. But I'm here today because she stopped keeping that bargain. Last week while running a work-related errand, she had her lunch in a bar, which led to a 3rd DUI, and this time she may go to jail. I've tried my best and it didn't work, so I feel like a loser who can't even protect his own family. What do I do now?

## Codependent Response

Can you imagine how this story would be viewed through the lens of Codependency? From that perspective Jack has unquestionably contributed to his wife's problem. In fact, he would be told that he was enabling and even encouraging it. He would also be told that he obviously had his own unresolved issues because he kept her drinking – perhaps related to his dad's alcoholism experienced when he was a kid. When approaching Jack from this perspective, he would be facing a clinical frame that describes him as enmeshed, enabling, and horribly Codependent. He would be told that his actions are a major contributor to Yvette's drinking. *Poor Jack, when will he understand that he is as sick as she is?*

## Prodependent Response

Through a Prodependent lens, Jack is viewed by the clinician as clever and highly resourceful. His actions are openly discussed and validated when seen through the lens of harm reduction. After all, he got his wife to stay sober during the day for 18 months. During that time, they had had steady income, no problems with the law, and kids who got home safely from school. Did Jack's solutions end his wife's battle with alcoholism? No. But is that because he is enabling, enmeshed, and has a deep unconscious desire to keep his wife sick? No. He didn't take more effective actions because he didn't know how.

Jack did the best he could to help keep his family going. It's not like he went to graduate school to study addiction! He did what he could to stop the repetition of the worst aspects of his wife's disease. In the addiction world, we even have a name for this, and it's called *harm reduction*. From a Prodependence perspective, we might even view him as a hero. He is in fact the very reason why there was a tolerable level of sanity and consistency in his and Yvette's home for a solid 18 months.

Does Jack need more help? Yes. Does he need help working through the early trauma wrought by *his* father's drinking to help his wife? No. At least not at this moment in time. What he does need from his counselor is compassion for his painful frustrations and validation for the steps he did take to keep family whole (whether those steps were useful in stopping the larger problem of alcoholism or not). And what he needs today – the reason he came to see you – is to get your professional help toward getting his wife sober and his family out of this mess as despite his best efforts he does not know how.

What Jack needs from us here is our direction, resources, hope, and support. How is it helpful, on any level, to ask him to look at his own history or his inability to set healthy boundaries? How do judgments, labels, and analytic concepts help him to get past his current crisis – as per Codependency? Obviously, they do not. And that is the reason Prodependence was created. We need not *blame the victims* of addicts. We need to support them.

## Basic Practices

Mental health professionals recognize that a caregiving loved one's lived experience of relationship stress, betrayal, or failure can be both highly traumatizing and disruptive in all areas of functioning. Because these individuals are often in this state of crisis when seeking therapeutic help, the earliest stages of treatment with a Prodependence-based therapist would:

### *Evaluate Client's Overall Condition by*

- Assessing for active mental illness/mood disorders.
- Assessing for level of client daily functioning – ADLs.
- Evaluating for any present physical or emotional danger to the client and family members (including the addict) – profound emotional or physical abuse, violence, child neglect, etc.
- Evaluating for any health or physical contributors to their problems – refer if needed.
- Providing mental health and addiction education toward helping the struggling person gain intellectual insight into their current circumstances.

- Assessing for current threats to the client's primary attachments, such as the loss of a family member to active addiction.
- Evaluating the degree to which this client has experienced similar related *adult* attachment trauma with this or other beloved individuals.
- Evaluating and validating all the ways this client has managed and reacted to the presenting life crisis (productive or not).

### *Applied Prodependence*

- Normalizing the client's changes in mood, functioning, self-care, and out-of-control feelings; explain these feelings/behaviors as typical of any/all persons who are neck-deep in an interpersonal crisis.
- Avoiding verbalizing any assumptions that past trauma bears a relationship to the current situation; instead, focus on the client's current reactivity to their current circumstances.
- If/when early trauma comes into the room, providing containment for those issues, using such past realities toward *shame reduction*. Note such issues for later discussion (if/when that time comes).
- Providing education and sources of further information on addiction, betrayal trauma, etc.
- Creating a deeper therapeutic alliance by normalizing the client's current experiences, feelings, and related actions as responses to the presenting crisis and not as something they have done wrong or something that is wrong with them.
- Telling the client there is nothing they could have done to prevent this.
- Telling the client there is nothing they did to make this happen.
- Telling the client that their support is a gift to the addict, but the addict's healing is ultimately the addict's work to do.
- Doing everything you can to connect the client to a community of support.
- Offering yourself as a resource to contact anytime. (Note: You don't have to answer the phone when the client calls, and you can tell them that. But the simple fact that you are listening is very reassuring.)

## The Initial Client Interview

Prodependence acknowledges – as stated – that early-life trauma that may not only be present in our client but is highly likely because nearly all of us, no matter how healthy, live with some degree of unresolved struggles from childhood. In the initial interview and early stages of treatment, however, Prodependence chooses to focus on the most current destabilizing events. The Prodependence model believes that it is counterproductive, shame-inducing, and possibly injurious to bring up or refer to the past until the presenting crisis is reasonably addressed and under control. We also believe – as stated – that such past trauma tends to reappear under the stress of living with an active addict (regression).

## Recognizing and Addressing Regression

It is common for clients in crisis to regress or fall back into thoughts, feelings, or behaviors from past trauma that left them feeling overwhelmingly fearful, out of control, or afraid. When any of us are in crisis, regression is a normative response. Thus, we should work to normalize it (via Prodependence) rather than exploring it (via Codependence).

Think about a child who stops bedwetting at age 4 but regresses back to it at 7 when experiencing a family crisis. Adults regress, too, but in more sophisticated ways. When we are overwhelmed or living in situations reminiscent of past traumatic events (abandonment, neglect, etc.), some of the feelings and behaviors that played out in the past can be come reactivated.

When this happens, it is best for therapists to utilize grounding and stabilizing interventions to help clients return to their previous level of functioning without shame or self-hatred. We do this while always reminding them that *feelings are not facts* and that we understand and accept their regression as a natural phenomenon. Generally, we are at our most effective when we guide our clients toward the kinds of tools and techniques that address what they feel and how they act in the present.

## Our Clinical Stance

The clinical underpinnings of the Prodependent-based model *encourage* us to be:

- Supportive and understanding.
- Empathic and nonjudgmental.
- Insightful and patient.
- Curious, not intrusive.
- Calm and open.
- Nurturing and engaged.
- Directive.
- Validating and reassuring.
- Focused on the problem at hand.
- Self-disclosing (when in the service of the client).
- Hopeful.
- Fully aligned with client goals.
- Active toward helping the client set boundaries.
- Aware of abuse, neglect, violence, etc.

With the Prodependence model, therapists can meet spouses, partners, and loved ones of addicts where they are, which is coming from a place of love and a desire for attachment. Rather than telling these folks they are an intrinsic part of the problem, we can acknowledge their hard work and the difficulties they've encountered in trying to help the addict. We can lead them toward caring for themselves as well as the addict, and we can help them provide loving assistance with better boundaries and an improved focus on self-care. All without blaming, shaming, or pathologizing.

The clinical qualities laid out by the Prodependence-based model *discourage* us from being:

- Deeply inquisitive about the past or any attempt to connect the clients' early-life past experiences to their present problems.
- Analytical by exploring any situation beyond the near or immediate present.
- Passive – that is, letting the clients struggle alone with their thoughts or feelings, and waiting for the clients to lead the conversation.
- Forceful by pushing clients to "get to work" and find their own resources.
- Emotionally distanced, as such clients need to feel your active compassion, attention, and immediate support.
- Vague or nondirective.
- Encouraging of the use of individual therapy as a sole source of healing, as such clients are best served by therapy combined with an external cohort of support.
- Intrusive by questioning the clients' motives or behaviors related to trying to help, rescue, or heal their troubled loved one.
- Judgmental of near any action the clients have taken in the service of healing their troubled loved one.
- Focused on the clients needing many years of therapy to deal with *their own* problems.
- A therapist who in any way labels or diagnoses someone who is highly emotionally reactive and/or in crisis (unless depression or another major mental health disorder is present and active).
- Unduly strict with our boundaries by only available at appointment-time. (Until the clients have identified or grown meaningful external resources, they need to count on us to be more responsive here than we might with a client who is not in crisis.)
- Focused on introductions concepts, models, books, or belief systems that may distract the clients from their present healing – that is, content on early-life trauma, any analysis of their relationship beyond the immediate crisis, introducing the concept of Codependency, etc.
- A clinician who primarily utilizes psychodynamic, Jungian, narrative, somatic, and other forms of noncrisis-related therapies in such situations.
- Viewing the clients as having their own addictive disorder to the addict themselves or to a loved one (beyond any potential active, unresolved substance or behavior addictions of their own).
- A "blank slate" thereby asking us to be opaque about ourselves and our intentions. These are situations that often require us to utilize appropriate forms of self-disclosure to reduce client shame and isolation. If

well-timed, self-disclosure (especially related to addiction) will lessen the clients' sense of being alone with the problem. An example follows:

> I want you to understand how deeply I relate to these experiences myself as a way to help with some of your shameful feelings and isolation. You see my own sister is an addict, and I clearly remember all the fear, pain, and anxiety that situation brought me and our whole family before she got finally sober. I strongly relate to how you feel. You are not alone. Just like you, I found it painful, even terrifying at times. Especially since I had no real control over getting her better, despite my love for her.

Prodependence suggests that part of restoring the clients' emotional, psychological, and situational balance involves constantly reminding ourselves how deeply and painfully they are being affected by interpersonal attachment trauma. These wounds may seem invisible or unconsciously held, but they are always there. Dr. Sue Johnson asserts that when the focus of treatment is non-pathologizing and flexible, an individual can focus on learning and growth through new experiences rather than attempting to remedy deficiencies or deficits.[1] Moreover, if an individual is experiencing a traumatic stress response to a crisis in their life, that person may present symptoms that mimic certain pathologies, such as personality disorders. It would therefore not be appropriate for a diagnosis to be assigned to that person until they are stabilized and have had time to process the events.

Similarly, Albert Roberts asserts there is an important difference between individuals responding to a crisis in a normative and adaptive way and those experiencing PTSD.[2] Thus, a diagnosis such as PTSD or a personality disorder should not be made hastily, before the initial shock has passed, or without proper assessments and evaluations. This is one of the reasons we have a provisional type diagnosis like Adjustment Disorders.

## Discourage Shame and Validate

Mental health and addiction professionals should also be aware of the tendency of caregiving loved ones of addicts to understandably blame themselves for the actions and behaviors of their troubled loved one. Here, the therapist's expressions and choice of words matter a great deal. Loved ones are already battling thoughts about what they could have and should have done better (remorse), often coupled with societal (and Codependency-based) blame for being enmeshed and for enabling their loved one's troubling behaviors. The language of Prodependence creates peace of mind simply by recognizing the client's pain and acknowledging the client's courageous efforts to save a crumbling connection.

Jesse Geller and Barry Farber agree that therapists must create a secure base, like in other meaningful relationships, from which the clients can examine and share their thoughts and feelings for the therapy to be most useful.[3] The authors state that the most useful therapeutic treatment begins with a supportive relationship with a clinician "who can create a no-judgment zone full of empathy and understanding.[4] Going back to Dr. Sue Johnson's work, she believes the right approach to therapy with this population can create safety while also providing a secure base from which the clients can explore difficult emotions and situations.[5]

Rose Barlow et al. suggest the most critical interventions in the earliest interactions with a client should focus on stabilization and fostering safety before addressing the actual trauma symptoms.[6] The work of Martin Dorahy et al. suggests a similar tactic, stating that since dissociation in treating complex trauma causes more distress than shame does, early interventions for this population should be focused on education and fostering a safe therapeutic bond.[7] This direction would include helping the individuals manage their responses to shame to better avoid withdrawal and avoidance in their relationship.

## Initial Client Interactions

The importance of initiating trauma-informed interventions before the clients embark on any complex intervention or specified program cannot be overstated. (A reminder here to the reader that the word "trauma" here is not meant to reference early childhood issues or any other past injuries that lie beyond the scope of addiction-focused crisis stabilization.) To this end, even before screening and assessment tools are utilized with such individuals, Denise Elliott et al. suggest that several things should be considered by the mental health provider:

- Any impairments to the clients' ability to trust the therapist.
- Any impairments to the patients gaining the support and insight available (panic attacks, suicidality, homicidal thoughts, physical illness, addiction, mood disorders, etc.).
- The clients' right to know the nature and purpose of the questions being asked.
- The potential emotional impact of the questions being asked.
- Giving the clients permission to not answer any question we pose to them.
- Allowing the clients to take or not take our recommendations.
- Clarity about the reason(s) for asking specific questions.[8]

When clients walk through the front door of a Prodependence-based therapist's office:

- The environment should be calm and inviting.
- The therapist should listen more than talk.
- When talking, the therapist should be curious, validating, and supportive, offering practical suggestions and direction.

- Information given to the clients should be easily understandable.
- Instructions given should be simple and tangible.

In all cases, therapists should mitigate the impact of ongoing interpersonal trauma and crisis by *allowing the clients to retain as much control as possible*. This means the therapist should involve the clients in all the decisions surrounding their treatment.

- *Therapist*: "I know you are in pain. I also know how out-of-control all of this feels, like no one is listening to you. And you are the sane one in the relationship. So here's a thought. Whatever you don't want to talk about, let me know and we will move on. If there's something I suggest that you don't like or want to take on just now, no problem. I am here to support you, not to leave you feeling more overwhelmed or out-of-control than when you arrived."

Additional therapeutic considerations include clearly explaining the rationale behind any question asked – making sure the clients are "in on" their treatment right from the start. This is the road toward a healthy and necessary therapeutic alliance.

- *Therapist*: "Would it be OK if I ask you some general questions about how your brother treats your parents? I am not trying to pry; I'm asking because I want to make sure that everyone living with your brother is physically and emotionally safe."

Counselors should also be attuned to the clients' level of trust. At times, the professional may give the clients the reins of the meeting (within limits), encouraging the clients to simply ask questions to gain clarity (and a sense of control).

- *Therapist*: "What things would you like for me to know about you today? I can see that you have a lot on your plate. If you feel like telling me more about the burdens you carry, maybe we can work together to lighten your load."

The therapist should also pay close attention to the tone of the words the clients use when describing their role in problem, working in real time to normalize *all their feelings about it*. When the clients start taking responsibility for issues that we can clearly see have been out of their control, we can simply reframe them as the best decisions they could make when living with such overwhelming circumstances.

- *Client*: "If I wouldn't have given my brother my car to use, maybe he wouldn't have been pulled over and arrested. I had a feeling I shouldn't but did it anyway."

- *Therapist*: "Well, that's one way of thinking about it. I wonder if we might consider another path. If you hadn't lent him your car, don't you think he would have harassed all his friends or your parents until he got someone else to lend him theirs? I think you should stop blaming yourself for your brother's addictive choices. Addicts are going to do what they want to do – one way or the other. His actions and decisions can never be your fault."

## Client Assessment

Early contact with near any client in a therapeutic setting, regardless of the presenting issue, involves evaluation and assessment, usually some form of standardized biopsychosocial Q&A. Traditionally, such assessments include information gathering in several different arenas, starting with general information, and then progressing to more specifics following what we learned from the standard, more general evaluations. Michael Kavan et al. believe that for clients who have experienced crisis to feel safe and navigate their future experiences successfully, it is critical that the clinician uses appropriate assessments and interventions.[9]

An essential element of early crisis intervention treatment – any good therapy, really – lies in our ability to provide a comprehensive assessment of the client beyond the basic biopsychosocial tools already familiar to most of us. Of course, a basic client evaluation is required as it points us generally in the right direction. If we wish to more deeply attune our work to "where the client is" in this situation, we are required to examine the effect of the active crisis of a loved one's addiction and how this is affecting their global functioning.

As a crisis-focused identification is a necessary assessment task, a sample Crisis Response Inventory, designed to be used in conjunction with a standard biopsychosocial and other relevant assessments, can be found in the Appendix in Chapter 6.

## Early Treatment Planning

Creating an effective treatment plan will include the goals of crisis treatment mentioned previously. The following elements should be included:

- Client information.
- Presenting complaint.
- Treatment summary.
- Treatment objectives.
- Treatment goals.
- Client strengths.

**Sample Treatment Plan**

| | |
|---|---|
| **CLIENT NAME** | Jane Smith |
| **DOB** | March 7, xxxx |
| **WORKING DIAGNOSIS** | Adjustment Disorder with Anxiety and Depression |
| **LIVING CIRCUMSTANCES** | Living with family of origin |
| **BIOLOGICAL SEX/AGE** | Female, 23 |
| **ANTICIPATED LENGTH OF TX** | 6 months |
| **ANTICIPATED REVISION OF TX PLAN** | 30 days |

**PRESENTING COMPLAINT**: Client is seeking treatment for her father's drug use, which has led to her parents constant fighting: slammed doors, plates being thrown, threats, and shouted obscenities all around.

Client states, "This is how it was when I left for college, but it's even worse now. I want to help them but I can't. I thought I could fix this or at least tolerate it, but I don't know how."

Client reports feeling lost, confused, and frustrated at her inability to effect meaningful change. She finds herself decreasingly able to fully function in her daily tasks. "It's not like I'm depressed. I actually feel good about having graduated school, and I'm looking forward to joining the military a year from now. But I'm here because over the past few weeks I find myself struggling to focus on much of anything. I'm just too upset."

**CLINICAL OVERVIEW**: Client is a 23-year-old female who resides with her parents in the family home, having graduated from college in June of xxxx. She lives with her parents and younger sister (who has Down syndrome). Her older married brother lives abroad. Client appears to be experiencing a reactive trauma response with related situational depression/anxiety. Client reports feeling overwhelmed and says this is directly related to her home life. Client reports that she is struggling to complete daily tasks and routines and that she has been isolating from family, friends, and other social situations. She reports having difficulty sleeping and getting herself out of the house.

**CLIENT STRENGTHS:** Client is intelligent, self-aware, and motivated toward healing. Client has a supportive family and friend network both through personal contacts and her church community.

**SHORT-TERM OBJECTIVES**: Educate about addiction, attachment loss, trauma, and self-care. Provide guidance and direction on healing from trauma. Offer active direction and support toward practicing self-care, grounding, and setting/maintaining effective boundaries. Provide resources where client might join a cohort of support (most likely Adult Children of Alcoholics (AcoA)). Continue to monitor for worsening symptoms of depression and anxiety.

Overall objectives include stress reduction, stabilization of internal dysregulation, return to healthy coping, and increased socialization to improve daily functioning and ego strength.

## TREATMENT GOALS

- Complete any mood disorder or related assessments.
- Participate in Families of Addicts or similar support group.
- Establish and utilize daily goals for balance and stabilization.
- Ascertain and reengage their own support community (safe family, friends, pastor, etc.).
- Evaluate client for agoraphobic and sleep related problems.
- Set and maintain effective family boundaries.
- Learn to acknowledge when they are dysregulated and introduce self-care and grounding techniques to calm such responses.

Client Signature       Date
Therapist Signature    Date

## Timing Is Everything

At times, we can feel compelled to help our clients become conscious of how prior abuse, trauma, neglect, and the like are influencing their current circumstances. When clients tell us this information, we often think it's time to *go there* with them. And in many circumstances, depending on clients' stability and goals, this can be an extraordinary rich path toward healing. But this is not a universal way of providing clinical work.

Prodependence therapists are advised to carefully observe and listen intently when treating the immediate interpersonal crisis, avoiding the temptation to spring into analytic or exploratory action. At all times, Prodependence-oriented therapists should *avoid* calling out, naming, and labeling every problem they observe. A well-trained and insightful therapist knows when to show their cards and when to keep them hidden. One of the best lessons that any mental health or addiction professional can learn is how to tolerate their desire to explore everything the client brings into the room the moment the client brings it in. If we see a lot of "stuff" that the client does not, *we can simply write it down*. We need to carefully choose the timing of such interventions, remembering that our goal is to normalize and stabilize and not to explore.

## Picking the Right Battles

Providing clients guidance to navigate through conflict with their troubled other will help with early stabilization and grounding. As the experience of a primary attachment rupture can create a fertile breeding ground for dissension, the clients' ability to discern between productive conflict and unwinnable battles empowers them to be more intentional about the battles they face. By encouraging boundary setting, social support, and self-care, we help them successfully maneuver through addiction-related conflicts.

- *Client*: "I can't believe that my wife is arguing with me about what color to paint the bathroom! This is just like her drinking. She can't see how her stubbornness is affecting everyone, so I'm not going to give in this time. I am going to paint our house whatever frickin' color I want."
- *Therapist*: "Even though your wants and needs often take a back seat to your wife's drinking, I'm pretty sure that you have a lot more pressing issues to handle right now than paint colors. How about this? When your wife is sober, and I know she will get there, there will be a day when you can paint the place together."

## Ambivalent Love: Hating and Loving at the Same Time

When we feel deep love and connection to another person, should they fail us or themselves in some deeply disturbing way – like becoming an opioid addict who steals money from the family to buy drugs – we hate that behavior. We hate them for doing it. And yet the years of our loving and being attached to them don't go away. So internal conflicts start to show up, and we find ourselves experiencing feelings of both love and hate at the same time.

For many caregivers and loved ones of addicts, these conflicting feelings can be confusing and alarming. Still, all of us can handle having two diametrically opposed feelings about the same situation, regardless of our circumstances. This is human. Thus, we can love someone and hate them at the same time. Just because someone left you *after* being increasingly abusive to you while you were together doesn't mean you are going to immediately stop being loving or being deeply attached to them. In the world of addiction, we often tell our clients, "Hate the behavior, not the person."

Naturally, people fear losing their relationships, so there can be a sense that it is not safe to disrupt the status quo of the relationship, despite not being totally happy with it. Even admitting a relationship may be experiencing difficulties feels terrifying enough for people to remain silent, minimize, or dismiss their ambivalent, mixed feelings. This can lead to people becoming stuck, continually focused on trying to avoid the inner discomfort they are experiencing rather than acknowledging and addressing it.[10]

By normalizing such feelings of ambivalent love, we help our clients find peace, within this confusing emotional duality. In fact, the integration of both emotions is a natural result of the healing journey. You can see one small example of this in the next statement, given by the caregiving husband of an opiate-addicted wife.

> When I look over at her sleeping, or holding our child, my heart is filled with love and gratitude. But at dinner time when she spills the food all over the table, zones out in front of the children, or simply forgets to join the family, I hate her. What is wrong with me?

What is wrong with this man? Nothing. Even though he himself feels broken and confused. Like any person, his emotions rise and fall according to circumstances. But not the inner connection that he shares with this wife. In this sense, we can think of long-term love by using a metaphor about the ocean. On the top, there can be choppy waters or calm, storms or sunshine, but regardless of what is happening on the surface, there are always deeply moving waters below. And those deeper currents are rarely affected by what is happening above.

Familial love (in all forms) is just like that. When someone we love is actively engaging in addictive behavior, we can love, hate, withdraw from, and move toward that person – all in the same afternoon. This can be viewed as our attempt to maintain deeper connections while life on the surface seems like an unpredictable mess.

## About Denial

The concept of client denial is widely acknowledged in psychotherapy as a defense. It is also relevant in Prodependent-based treatment when understood from a safety perspective. In other words, clients often deny certain elements of their situation due to its complex and traumatic nature. When addictions are present, people can deny what is happening right in front of them to lessen the day-to-day impact of their experience. They often make choices consciously or unconsciously, helpful or not, that allow them to look away from their truth to survive it. Thus, we can expect loved ones of addicts to minimize, rationalize, externalize, and otherwise distort the details of their situation – all to make it seem more bearable and less impactful.

When we point out a deeply connected partner or family member's cognitive distortions (as opposed to our work with addicts), we do so very slowly, starting with the most concerning issues, for example, verbal abuse and highly problematic behaviors (on either side).

When working with addicts, confronting denial head-on, or nearly head-on, is often the best path to help them get sober. But in the case of caregivers and loved ones, a Prodependent therapist can and should be more patient. We do this with the understanding that denial is always a self-protective mechanism (a defense) that typically corrects itself in smaller and larger ways as the client experiences safety via our supportive alliance combined with the care of loving community and family others. But, as stated earlier, we are required to directly confront patients' denial if their distorted thoughts and related actions have caused them to tolerate abuse or to act it out themselves.

## About Rage

Rage is a mixture of many different intense emotions (anger, fear, sadness, etc.) felt all at the same time. It is an explosive and hurtful expression of feelings – whether it is turned toward others or the self – that can be quite damaging. When we experience rage, we are not intellectually present or grounded. We are fully emotionally engaged, with little ability to make healthy, rational decisions. Once again, this is because the limbic (feeling) part of our brain has hijacked our ability to think rationally, calmly, and clearly.

If client is experiencing bouts of rage, the therapist should provide education on what is happening by raising awareness while helping the client gain the tools and interventions required to de-escalate.

As previously stated, *physical abuse is never acceptable* and verbal abuse is to be avoided whenever possible. In such situations, the client is well served when we utilize cognitive behavioral methods. Perhaps we help them create a step-by-step rage-awareness plan or teach them about time-outs. We might also use verbal or written contracts and agreements, our goal being to raise our clients' awareness of how they feel and what they need to do to keep from boiling over. Sadly, sometimes the best we can do is to help someone walk away (long-term or short-term) from abusive situations.

## About Violence and Abuse

When active addictions are present in a relationship, it is not uncommon for either party to end up using abusive and/or violent language and behaviors. This can happen when any of us feels profoundly unstable and emotionally dysregulated. Addicts, in particular, can be mean, violent, angry, irritable, dismissive, and all the rest when using. Spouses too can throw plates, hit, yell, slam doors, and threaten in ways not typical for them.

Examples of abuse or violence within an addictive (or any) relationship can include:

- Physical acts of aggression.
- Repeatedly telling another that they are worthless, don't deserve to live, etc.

- Threatening the life, safety, or health of another.
- Threatening to take away kids or other meaningful others.
- Explaining the situation to children to gain their sympathy.
- Blame, manipulation, and gaslighting.
- Attempting to gain excessive control over another person.
- Exposing children to adult aggression (verbal or physical).
- Sexual violations (no consent, etc.).
- Undermining the other's goals, plans, or self-esteem.
- Breaking things, throwing things, punching walls, and otherwise frightening or threatening the other with violence.

If we as therapists learn of this type of behavior, we must intervene on one or both parties. First and foremost, we must provide the kind of safety-first tools and suggestions that will keep all parties safe and focused on the problem at hand. To this end, we can assist our clients in developing and implementing a plan for physical and/or emotional distancing. Other times, we might counsel that it is best that one or the other person simply leave the situation altogether, at least for a time. When violence and abuse are recognized by the therapist, the client's safety (or the addict's) takes priority over all other therapeutic interventions or activities. And, of course, should we hear of potentially life-threatening behaviors, we are ethically (and legally) required to report these issues to the proper authorities.

## Identifying and Treating Shame Versus Guilt

The presence of shame (formerly referred to as "toxic shame") is a common phenomenon for all humans. This is especially true in those who are dealing with embarrassing or shameful (to them) situations like active addiction. Brené Brown describes shame as "the intensely painful feeling or experience of believing that we are flawed and therefore unworthy of love and belonging."[11] Individuals with an active interpersonal crisis often experience deeply negative underlying assumptions about themselves, and are therefore more prone to feeling flawed and shameful. Brown states that although shame is something all human beings will experience, the need to appear put together on the outside to avoid being defined by even one shameful experience is a sincere challenge.[12] This can be especially true for families and loved ones of addicts and similarly struggling individuals, as betrayal and often public struggles may carry intense levels of disgrace.

Common shameful beliefs held by loved ones of addicts include:

- Something is wrong with me, that's why this happened.
- I'll never be good enough for anyone.
- I am not worthy of loving.
- I don't deserve to get my needs met.

- Nothing I do and no one I love will give me a happy life.
- Nothing I do makes any difference.
- I'm not worthy of a healthy partner.
- If people could see who I really am, they wouldn't love or care about me.
- I can't trust other people to meet my needs.
- This kind of relationship is all I deserve.
- I was a bad parent, which is what led to all of this.
- Considering how I have lived my life, I probably deserve this.
- If I had been more loving, more available, more... this wouldn't have happened.

Shame is invited in when friends, family, and others ask, "Why are you staying in this relationship?" or say, "I never thought she was right for you." When we tell caregivers and other loved ones of addicts that something is wrong with them for being or staying in this relationship, we leave them doubting themselves in unhealthy ways. When we challenge their choice to stay around to help or, worse, tell them that they are Codependent (and thus something is wrong with them), we hurt them.

No matter how well-intended, this is not the way to support anyone. It's like abandoning them to thoughts of not being worth loving or not deserving to get their needs met in any relationship based on their own core shortcomings. In addition to the stigma that addiction itself brings, such loved ones may themselves have a history of early-life shame that flares up due to their current out-of-control fears (again regression). Prodependence doesn't seek to explore their shame; it does, however, seek to normalize such understandable feelings by reframing them as feeling guilt and responsibility for the problem.

## The Impact of Shame

Shame can affect every aspect of a relationship and fuel an already hostile environment by perpetuating feelings of low self-worth and a general lack of self-compassion. This can make it difficult for caregiving loved ones to be present with their own emotions and the emotions of others.

As previously stated, when people in pain can join a live (or online) cohort of others in a similar situation, this often helps counteract debilitating feelings of shame. Most often, their healing work becomes more effective when completed in a healthy group setting. Brené Brown states that an individual's sense of connection and strength are enhanced when they can receive non-shaming empathy from other via shared compassion and support.

A Prodependent therapist will recognize the impact of shame that accompanies addiction. Assisting caregivers in understanding and challenging shame-based distortions is essential to their healing. By challenging and confronting their negative beliefs, we clear a path toward their becoming gentler with themselves. This, in turn, can make receiving support, engaging in self-care, and engaging in other healthy behaviors feel more doable.

Possible shame-challenging responses include the following:

- It doesn't feel good to fail, but I am not supposed to be perfect.
- Even though feeling less-than is familiar, I am not the only one who has felt that way.
- It hurts to not feel loved sometimes, but that doesn't mean I'm not lovable.
- It is difficult when others let me down, but thankfully I can meet many of my own needs.
- It breaks my heart when I feel betrayed, but I am brave enough to keep trying.
- I didn't cause my loved one's addiction. Nothing I have ever done or said caused it or could have prevented it from happening.
- Whether I loved the addict in the right way or not, the addict's choices are not about me and never were.
- It's OK to feel terrible about what I am facing, but it's not OK to beat myself up about it.

## Differential Diagnosis

### *Physical Health*

It is a sad truth that clients, when in a family crisis like addiction, will often neglect the most basic forms of self-care due to a near singular focus on helping their addicted loved one. Upon interview, it is not unusual to learn that such clients have not been to a dentist, eye doctor, or had a thorough physical exam in many years. Some will present with prior or newly evolved health problems that have long gone unchecked or unaddressed like heart disease, diabetes, and the like. It is understandable that those living with the chronic stress of addiction may also have preexisting, seemingly resolved immune-related health concerns like MS or IBS escalate or reappear sometimes years after their seeming resolution.

There may be times when a client presents with an accompanying diagnosis that may take priority over or further complicate the existing crisis. These could include underlying medical, developmental, or physical conditions such as the following:

- Thyroid disease.
- Hormone disorders.
- Autism spectrum disorders.
- Developmental disorders.
- Chronic or terminal disease.
- Physical or cognitive disabilities.
- Pregnancy.
- Diabetes (and other chronic illnesses that require ongoing focus and attention).
- Unresolved or recent physical losses.

Part of our ongoing evaluation and relationship with our clients is to learn about such issues, while actively encouraging better physical care. Keep in mind that *self-care* is not always about meditation, attending support groups, taking time off, journaling, massage, and yoga. Self-care starts with the basics of proper rest, eating, and exercise while actively monitoring any active health concerns. Note, too, that *it is a primary responsibility* of all addiction and mental health professionals to ensure that any potential physical health concerns are evaluated and treated (if necessary) before we begin to accurately diagnose and plan treatment. Without such awareness and actions, we can easily misdiagnose our clients, thus providing therapies that are ineffective or misaligned with client need.

Ethical, well-trained clinicians must be able to differentiate common presenting issues like grief, loss, sadness, anger, and chronic disappointment from more profound concerns like depression, bipolar disorders, and psychosis, which require treatment methods that are beyond our skill set. Healthy, well-rounded counselors must always be open to seeking out the feedback and direction from other professionals should they not be well versed in the signs and symptoms of specific mental health disorders. It is our strong belief that clinicians providing direct care to clients must know their own clinical strengths and vulnerabilities to best serve their clients or refer them to other professionals.

Physical health concerns will lead us to encourage doctors' visits and appropriate, related medical care, while profound mental health issues are best evaluated by a well-trained psychiatrist or mental health professional. There are several national nonprofit agencies providing support toward dealing with mental illness in a loved one, the largest among which are NAMI (the National Alliance on Mental Illness) and the NIMH (the National Institute of Mental Health). Such organizations offer needed direction, tools, and insight for families and loved ones in those situations.

Treating therapists should always assess for physical health concerns in the initial intake interview. This may include working in tandem with other providers to guide the healing path in the most ethical and effective ways for the client.

### *Mental Health*

While the focus of this training guide is to lead therapists and counselors toward more effective, strength-based (Prodependent) ways for families to heal from addiction, there are primary – sometimes related – issues that professionals are also responsible to identify and address. Beyond assessing for physical health issues, leading the pack is the challenge of mental illness in the addict or loved ones being treated. Despite our focus toward evolving more compassionate forms of strength-based, addictive healing in the family, there can always be unexpected impediments to the process related to underlying mental illness, the activation of past trauma, or both. Just as you can't eat a meal until it is cooked, nor can we carry out the themes and practices of Prodependence while our clients or their addicted loved one struggles with underlying issues that can delay or even prevent their growth.

While there are no universal mental health concerns that can be identified among the families and spouses of addicts, common sense tells us that living in seemingly unresolvable, chronically painful situations can lead to situational or chronic mood disorders like depression and anxiety. Experience tells us that profound stress and hypervigilance experienced over time can exacerbate past abuse and trauma, and/or preexisting mental health concerns like personality-based, psychotic, delusional and/or addictive problems. In such cases, we are likely to see a range of related presenting problems like co-occurring addictions (food, substance abuse), panic attacks, relationship dysfunction, poor sleep, inability to follow through, suicidality, memory problems, and the like. In such cases, we may find ourselves referring to psychiatrists or other experts to further support and clarify our work.

## Complex Cases

Comorbid psychological disorders should always be considered when initiating any therapeutic treatment for this population. Some examples of these disorders include the following:

- Personality disorders.
- Bipolar and related disorders.
- Depressive disorders
- Anxiety disorders.
- Obsessive-compulsive and related disorders.
- Dissociative disorders.
- Schizophrenia spectrum and other psychotic disorders.
- Neurodevelopmental disorders.
- Trauma and stressor-related disorders.
- Substance-related and addictive disorders.
- Somatic symptom and related disorders.
- ADHD.
- Sleep-wake disorders.
- Neurocognitive disorders.

If a client presents any of these disorders in conjunction with the current crisis, steps should be taken to first assess how such disorders may affect or otherwise complicate their situation and their emotional healing. Referrals and evaluations may be needed before we can proceed with our part of the work. There are times when we need to turn our focus to the treatment of the accompanying disorder before Prodependence work can effectively take place. It is up to us to find the delicate balance between existing pathologies and current client needs when initiating Prodependent psychological care.

## Useful Treatment Modalities

Part four of this book provides a series of treatment exercises that we find effective, from a Prodependence perspective, when working with loved ones of addicts. The exercises we provide arise from and work well in conjunction with numerous existing therapeutic modalities. Although this is not an exhaustive list, the following well-established modalities can enhance Prodependent-based treatment.

- Cognitive behavioral therapy (CBT): Because CBT is a short-term goal-oriented therapeutic modality that challenges the clients' thought processes and behavioral patterns, it can help them manage their stressful situation and difficulties in their relationship.

    ○ *Client:* "I can't be the right parent for this kid. She is so difficult, and I just don't have what it takes to keep dealing with her destructive behavior."

    ○ *Therapist:* "I would like you to make a list of all of the things you have done to help your daughter and put a checkmark next to the ones that you feel have worked in some way."

- Dialectical behavioral therapy (DBT): DBT can assist the clients who are struggling with emotional pain by helping them learn to better tolerate their distress.

    ○ *Client:* "My life is falling apart and there is nothing I can do about it. I feel like my head and heart are going to explode! If my boyfriend doesn't stop acting out sexually, I don't know what I am going to do!"

    ○ *Therapist:* "I can understand why you are so upset. Sometimes, as hard as it is, we have to find a way to refocus on the things we can change instead of the things we can't. I want to teach you some mindfulness exercises that will help when you are feeling overwhelmed. If you are willing, it might be useful to make a daily journal entry defining how you feel and why – something concrete to bring me so we can work on this together."

- Group therapy: Because loving someone with an addiction can be so isolating, participating in group therapy can help normalize the clients' suffering and increase their feelings of support and encouragement. Group participation can also help them identify their feelings and needs while also providing a safe place to express them. Such groups can be viewed more as gently moderated support groups rather than group therapy involving confrontation or explorations of the past.

    ○ *Client:* "It seems like I sit day after day wondering what bad thing my husband will do next to break my heart and don't have anyone to talk to about it. It feels like I must be the only one going through this."

    ○ *Group member:* "I can totally relate to what you are saying. There was no way I was going to tell my family or friends about my husband's bad choices. I didn't want everyone to hate him, I just needed to be able to talk to someone who could understand what I was going through and not judge either of us. Once I found some people who were in the same situation as me, I found myself feeling better."

- Eye movement desensitization and reprocessing (EMDR): EMDR is a psychotherapeutic intervention proven effective for the treatment of trauma (including post-traumatic stress disorder) by working with the circuitry in the brain to reduce the intensity of distressing emotions. Since relationship crises are a form of trauma, EMDR can be effective with loved ones of addicts.

  ○ *Therapist:* "From what you describe, every time you are faced with this or a similar situation, you have a panic attack. You find yourself unable to think clearly or function. This kind of very strong reaction can be more of an automatic brain response than something related to the problems at hand. I think doing some EMDR may help reduce some of these disabling experiences, thereby helping you maintain your sanity whatever the addict might say or do."

- Art therapy: Art therapy can enrich the client's healing journey through various creative processes. It can help with self-esteem, self-awareness, and emotional resilience while promoting insight, enhancing social skills, and reducing and resolving conflicts. Examples of art therapy include the following:

  ○ Drawing.
  ○ Painting.
  ○ Music.
  ○ Body movement.

- Journaling: Asking clients to use writing to express and identify their thoughts and feelings can often be more effective than talking. Writing can help clients organize experiences and access more specific details of events. Writing can also create safety in the therapeutic process by somewhat limiting the client's level of vulnerability to the traumatic event(s). Today's technology allows us access to a journal 24/7 via phones and tablets. Therefore, clients can write down whatever they feel, whenever they feel compelled to do so.

  ○ *Therapist:* "I would like you to take some time to write down your thoughts and feelings after each of our sessions in a journal. Don't worry about saying things just right or about the structure. Just freely express whatever comes to mind. The simple act of writing your thoughts down can help you to be less reactive and more objective."

- Somatic therapies: Somatic therapy is a form of body-centered therapy that looks at the connection of mind and body and utilizing both talk and physical therapies for holistic healing. In addition to talk therapy, somatic therapy practitioners use mind-body exercises and other physical techniques to help release the pent-up tension that is negatively affecting your physical and emotional well-being. The following are examples of mindfulness or somatic-based interventions:

  ○ Breathing exercises.
  ○ Guided imagery.

- ◦ Body scanning.
- ◦ Focusing on nature.
- ◦ Creative visualization.
- ◦ Yoga.
- ◦ Meditation.

Prodependence-oriented therapists are invited to explore these and other modalities in conjunction with the specific exercises we provide, recognizing that different clients will respond to different techniques. Better still, clients can provide feedback about what resonates and what does not, further empowering them as individuals while strengthening the therapeutic alliance.

## Defining the End of an Interpersonal Crisis

An addiction-related interpersonal/attachment crisis is over when one or two of the following occur:

1. The addict is fully in remission (sobriety). They are no longer using or acting out, and they have stable support and have made ongoing healing their priority. At that point, our work will refocus onto long-term stabilization, considerations of how to work with relapses, and resources for ongoing support.
2. Sometimes a loved one's relationship with the struggling individual is not destined to last. Regardless of the reason for the relationship ending, the client's work will then refocus onto grief, role identification, support, and direction while validating their life choices. Again our goal is here and now until the client has moved through their grief.

Note: Following either or both of the above circumstances our client may choose to leave therapy because they view their problem as resolved. Unless there is an emergent or unforeseen problem, at this point we validate their choices and work toward closure. That said, it is never our job to force a client to stay, nor is it our job to explain the mistake they are making by leaving so quickly. Instead, we ensure that they have sufficient external support should they need it. We encourage (and schedule) a few follow-up sessions to check up with them over time. As always we reinforce the idea that our door is always open should they need help in the future and then help define when such help might be needed.

## Crisis Resolution Is Our Focus!

Although it would be ideal if a therapist could see monumental improvements in all areas of the client's life and functioning, it is best to manage these expectations. Individual situations are so varied, with such diverse levels of crisis, that the outcomes or treatment will vary widely from person to person.

That said, the interventions and skills employed in the Prodependence model are intended to help stabilize the client's crisis responses and create an environment for continued healing and growth, and this improvement should be apparent over time. There are not, however, distinct stages of healing in the earliest weeks of Prodependence treatment; rather, there are indicators of stabilization to which the therapist should be attuned.

The following is a potential list of changes and observations that will assist the therapist in measuring client progress and healing:

- A reduction of active fear and helplessness (i.e., a reduction in limbic/trauma responses).
- An increasing ability to self-soothe via social support, mindfulness, and other grounding techniques.
- Recognition of their own emotional overwhelm and knowing what they need to do to handle it.
- Involvement in a reliable community of support.
- Reduced shame as the clients refocus away from seeing themselves as part of the problem, shifting instead to seeing themselves as part of the solution.
- Ability to challenge negative cognitions and beliefs with compassionate alternatives.
- Ability to adjust daily patterns and maintain greater balance.
- Shifting toward healthy boundaries with the addict.
- Insight into feelings and related reactivity.
- Prioritization of self-care.
- Awareness of and processing of grief related to the addiction and relationship losses.
- Internalization of the fact that they did not cause the addiction and it is not their job to fix it.
- Emotional stabilization.

The clinical framework, underlying belief systems, and refocus of the clients' problem(s) are what delineates Prodependence from other models designed to help caregivers and loved ones of addicts. We deeply believe that this new perspective will allow mental health professionals to effectively utilize attachment-focused healing for those facing the ravages of a loved one's addiction.

By offering a fully new way to view and treat loved ones of addicts – a 180-degree turn from prior pathology-focused work – we encourage every counselor to provide more strength-based, non-pathological, here-and-now support to this long-misunderstood population. We have experienced this new model in our practices as a more effective and kinder way to help our clients survive this type of interpersonal crisis. We hope that this new and evolving paradigm leads to the kind or self-efficacy and self-forgiveness that will help loved ones of addicts to successfully maneuver not just through their current crisis but any potential future crisis.

# Notes

1. Johnson, S. M. (2004). *The practice of emotionally focused couples therapy* (2nd ed.). Taylor & Francis.
2. Roberts, A. R. (2002). Assessment, crisis intervention, and trauma treatment: The integrative ACT intervention model. *Brief Treatment and Crisis Intervention, 2*(1), 1–22. https://doi.org/10.1093/brief-treatment/2.1.1
3. Geller, J. D., & Farber, B. A. (2015). Attachment style, representations of psychotherapy, and clinical interventions with insecurely attached clients. *Journal of Clinical Psychology, 71*(5), 457–468. https://doi.org/10.1002/jclp.22182
4. Weiss, R. (2018). *Prodependence: Moving beyond Codependency.* Health Communications, Inc.
5. Johnson, S. M. (2019). *Attachment theory in practice.* The Guilford Press.
6. Barlow, M. R., Goldsmith Turrow, R. E., & Gerhart, J. (2017). Trauma appraisals, emotion regulation difficulties, and self-compassion predict posttraumatic stress symptoms following childhood abuse. *Child Abuse and Neglect, 65*, 37–47. https://doi.org/10.1016/j.chiabu.2017.01.006
7. Dorahy, M. J., Corry, M., Shannon, M., Webb, K., McDermott, B., Ryan, M., & Dyer, K. F. W. (2013). Complex trauma and intimate relationships: The impact of shame, guilt and dissociation. *Journal of Affective Disorders, 147*, 72–79. https://doi.org/10.1016/j.jad.2012.10.010
8. Elliott, D. E., Bjelajac, P., Fallot, R. D., Markoff, L. S., & Reed, B. G. (2005). Trauma-informed or trauma-denied: Principles and implementation of trauma-informed services for women. *Journal of Community Psychology, 33*(4), 461–477. https://doi.org/10.1002/jcop.20063
9. Kavan, M., Guck, T., & Barone, E. (2006). A practical guide to crisis management. *American Family Physician, 74*(7), 1159–1164.
10. https://welldoing.org/article/feel-ambivalent-about-relationship
11. Brown, B. (2012). *Daring greatly.* Penguin Random House.
12. Brown, B. (2010). *The gifts of imperfection.* Hazelden Publishing.

# Section 4

# The Workbook

## Introduction

The following workbook provides the mental health professional with Prodependence-oriented exercises to utilize with loved ones of addicts in individual and group therapy. These exercises are split into five sections – based on the five primary goals of crisis treatment, as outlined earlier in this book. As a reminder, these goals are the following:

1. Normalization and Mitigation of Crisis.
2. Support and Connection.
3. Basic Information and Education.
4. Hope.
5. Healing.

The 22 exercises in this workbook are simple and straightforward in nature, intended to be a starting point for this specialized clientele, and to be used primarily in the earliest stages of treatment – when the client is *still in crisis* and unable to process and implement anything too complicated. Thus, for the most part, these tasks are geared toward the client's physiological, emotional, and behavioral stabilization.

This workbook is ultimately designed for use within both individual and group therapy for partners and other loved ones of addicts. In our experience, group therapy is especially effective, as group members can hold one another accountable and provide feedback to one another based on observations and personal experience. Certain exercises, of course, lend themselves to further examination and processing in individual sessions.

There is not a prescribed length of time for this "program," nor is there a structured "lesson plan" for use. We encourage you, as therapists, to assign these exercises to your clients as appropriate. Yes, we have placed them in a specific order, with that order being organized by treatment goals. But depending on the client and the client's specific needs on any given day, this order may change. We leave such decisions up to you, the therapist. That said, we recommend that exercises focused on Normalization and Mitigation be taught first, as they help to create stability while building coping skills that are useful when completing and processing later work.

It is possible that some loved ones of addicts, especially those who are already familiar with the concept of Prodependence through Dr. Rob Weiss's initial book on this topic or the newly formed Prodependence Anonymous self-help program, will pick up this clinical guide, find this workbook section, and attempt to work the exercises on their own. In such cases, we strongly encourage these individuals to share their work with supportive others, asking for feedback and support as needed – and even when they think it is not needed. Simply stated, developing a habit of reaching out to supportive, empathetic others for help with one's problems is, in and of itself, Prodependent. And learning to be Prodependent is the whole purpose of this book.

Our hope, however, is that these exercises will be undertaken with the guidance of a Prodependence-oriented therapist in conjunction with both individual and group therapy.

Please note: The 22 exercises contained herein are not unique to Prodependence. They are purposefully neither new nor groundbreaking. As therapists, you are likely familiar with many of them, and you may have assigned versions of them to clients in the past. If so, we applaud you, but we also ask you to consider using the versions in this workbook rather than older ones. We ask this as we have written this workbook using the updated language of Prodependence, with a clear focus on supportive, empathetic interdependence.

Each exercise has a brief introduction explaining its purpose and how to work it. We have also provided numerous sample answers to help clients understand what they're supposed to do, and to help open their minds to responses they might not otherwise consider.

Finally, we wish to acknowledge that this workbook is not the be-all, end-all of treating loved ones of addicts. As stated earlier, we believe these exercises will be incredibly helpful in the early stages of treatment, but even then, they should be only part of the treatment regimen. You, as the therapist, will need to continually evaluate and assess the needs of your clients and adjust treatment accordingly – not only moving around in the workbook as appropriate, but adding other exercises and methodologies that you believe will be helpful – EMDR, somatic work, psychodrama, family sculpting art therapy, CBT, DBT, and more. The more grounded, varied, and sophisticated your approach, the more successful you are likely to be.

## Workbook Structure

Stage 1: Normalization and Mitigation of Crisis

- Relationship Trauma
- Stabilizing Tools
- Mindful Walking Meditation
- Bonus Skill: 5-4-3-2-1 Grounding

- Relaxation Breathing Exercises
- The Self-Compassionate Eye

Stage 2: Support and Connection

- Identifying Your Unmet Needs
- Meeting Your Needs
- List of Support
- Call to Courage

Stage 3: Basic Information and Education

- Safety-Seeking Checklist
- Balance – the Rowboat
- Shame Prevention Plan
- Loss Inventory
- Anger Inventory

Stage 4: Hope

- The Grief Letter
- My Rights Manifesto
- Loving Support
- Personal Serenity Mantra

Stage 5: Healing

- Healthy Boundaries
- Letting Go
- Reflection Artwork
- Healthy Living Plan

## Stage 1: Normalization and Mitigation of Crisis

When individuals seeking therapeutic help are in a relationship crisis, such as we see when loved ones of the clients are addicted, the clients want, more than anything, to feel better. They want their life back. They want to resume the past thoughts, feelings, and activities available to them before their lives started spinning out of control. The following five exercises (plus a bonus skill) are designed to help with this process.

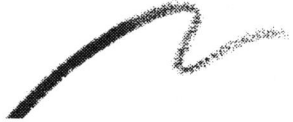

## Exercise 1
## Relationship Trauma

The disconnection that happens when a family member is addicted can feel devastating to a caregiving loved one. This experience of relationship trauma feels similar to other types of trauma. For example, trauma wrought by addiction can cause traumatic stress reactions, where specific parts of the brain are activated. In particular, your brain may go into a fight/flight/freeze response. As a result, you might experience an uncomfortable free fall of negative thoughts and emotions. This does not mean there is anything wrong with you. It simply means you are having a painful (and relatively normal) response to a threatening situation.

Wherever you are in your relationship with your struggling loved one, it will benefit you to pay close attention to your body and the emotional signals that indicate an attachment trauma wound is being activated. This way, you can use your tools and take the steps you have learned to get through those difficult moments.

The following is a list of common trauma symptoms. This is not an exhaustive list; it is a starting place to help you identify what has happened. Circle the symptoms that you are currently experiencing or have experienced in the past.

Dizziness
Irritability
Unwanted thoughts
Lightheadedness
Trembling
Hostility
Sweating
Heart racing
Headaches
Social withdrawal
Nausea
Argumentative
Consistent feelings of impending doom
Defensiveness
Inability to concentrate
Self-destructive behaviors

Tunnel-vision
Quick and drastic mood changes
Extreme anxiety
Impulsive behaviors
Depression
Substance or alcohol abuse
Inability to control reactive thoughts
Sexual problems
Inability to maintain healthy close relationships
Dissociative symptoms
Hopelessness
Feeling permanently damaged
Intrusive and frightening dreams/nightmares
Other:
Other:
Other:

What relationship injuries have you experienced?

*Example: My husband has repeatedly chosen alcohol over me, our relationship, and our family. He has been fired from multiple jobs and has failed in his promise to provide for the family while I take care of our home and children.*

1. _____

2. _____

3. _____

4. _____

5. _____

6. _____

7. _____

_____

_____

_____

8. _____

_____

_____

_____

9. _____

_____

_____

_____

10. _____

_____

_____

_____

What has it been like for you to experience these injuries?

*Example: I am totally devastated by what has happened. I can't believe this is my life and that I'm in the situation I am in because of someone else's choices. I just want to be loved and count on a future free of this kind of pain and hurt.*

_____

_____

_____

_____

_____

How have you tried to manage, fix, or repair the damage from these injuries?

*Example: I have tried so hard to help my husband see how his bad choices are affecting him and everyone around him. I have made appointments for him, checked in on him day and night, and talked until I am blue in the face. Nothing ever seems to help.*

_____

_____

_____

_____

_____

What hopes and dreams for your relationship were dashed when these injuries happened?

*Example: I have always dreamed of being able to talk openly with my husband about my feelings without him being defensive and angry.*

_____

_____

_____

_____

_____

What negative emotions and trauma responses have you felt since this happened?

*Example: I have not been able to sleep more than three hours a night without getting woken up with thoughts about my husband's drinking and his other bad behaviors.*

_____

_____

_____

_____

_____

What longing for connection with the addict have you kept to yourself because it is too embarrassing or painful?

*Example: I wish I could have a healthy sexual relationship with my husband. But instead, our sexual interaction leaves me feeling used. I would feel really embarrassed to tell anyone about that.*

_____

_____

_____

_____

_____

If there could be an ideal future outcome, what would that be?

*Example: My husband getting sober from his addiction to alcohol and learning to deal with his struggles in a healthier way.*

_____

_____

_____

_____

_____

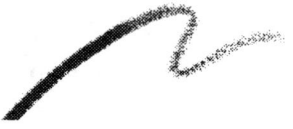

**Exercise 2**
**Stabilizing Tools**

Unfortunately, when you are in close relationship with an addict, negative thoughts and feelings are unavoidable. You will see or hear something, or the addict will do something that pushes you toward the chaos and stress of addiction. Often, this will happen with zero warning at a time when everything seems OK or even good. You're just hanging around having a good day, minding your own business, and bam! Suddenly, your fight/flight/freeze response is activated. Occasionally, you won't even know what triggered this response; you'll just find yourself in the middle of the insanity again.

These periodic flashes of chaos are deeply unsettling even in the best of circumstances; doubly so when you are already feeling overwhelmed with life, thanks to your loved one's addiction. The good news is that you needn't stay in this activated, reactionary state (where you are likely to behave in ways you might later regret). Instead, you can turn to the stabilizing tools discussed next (and throughout this workbook) as a way to calm your elevated emotions.

The tools examined here (and later) are ongoing skills you can use throughout your healing journey and throughout your life. We have divided them by categories – physical, personal, relational, and spiritual – to place them in real-world context. Please understand these are just a few of the coping skills available to loved ones of addicts. The list we've provided here is a great start but hardly the full toolkit; you'll want to develop other skills as your healing journey progresses.

*Physical*: Things you need to care for your physical body and physical health.

- *Get moving*: Stand up, walk around, stretch, etc.
- *Take a break*: Take a power nap, watch a video, read a daily inspiration, etc.
- *Breathe*: Close your eyes and slowly breathe in and out for a few minutes.
- *Time out*: Walk away (temporarily) from what you are doing and relax or do something else.
- *Exercise*: Go to the gym or go for a walk or run.
- *Get outside*: Do something outside like yardwork, walking the dog, sitting in the shade, etc.

*Personal*: Needs that address your feelings, growth, and what is most meaningful to you.

- *Healthy distraction*: Focus on something other than what is bothering you.
- *Thought topping*: Stop the negative thought you are focusing on and think about something positive.
- *Self-compassion messages*: Take a moment to say something kind to yourself.
- *Give yourself permission*: Tell yourself, "I can stop what I am doing right now," or, "It's OK to rest."
- *Have a laugh*: Put on a movie that makes you laugh.
- *Play*: Get out a hobby and work on it, go outside and play kickball with your kids, etc.
- *HALT*: HALT is an acronym for Hungry, Angry/Anxious, Lonely, and Tired. Loved ones of addicts must learn to ask themselves these basic questions about self-care: When is the last time I ate? Did I get enough sleep last night? Is there some conflict in my life that I need to resolve? Would a few minutes spent talking with someone who understands me help me to feel better? More often than not, a catnap, a candy bar, or a five-minute phone conversation will greatly diminish your negative thinking.

*Relational*: Things you need to build secure and stable connections with loved ones and others.

- *Phone call or text*: Call a friend and let them know what you are feeling.
- *Spend time with someone*: Go get coffee with a friend or colleague.
- *Serve*: Find someone in need and provide help to them.
- *Reach out for support*: If you're in a therapy group, support group, or 12-step recovery group, reach out to another member and chat for a few minutes.
- *Bookend potential triggers*: You can arrange to "bookend" potentially triggering events with phone calls to a supportive friend. During the "before" call, you commit to keeping a level head and relinquishing the need to control. The "after" call provides an opportunity to discuss what happened, what feelings came up, and what you might need to do differently next time.

*Spiritual*: Needs that are connected to your intrinsic value and spiritual self — as you define it.

- *Meditate*: Find a quiet and safe place to close your eyes and breathe.
- *Listen to music*: Turn on your favorite song or album and enjoy the music.
- *Read*: Grab an interesting book and read for a few minutes.
- *Journal*: Get out a notebook and write down your thoughts and feelings.
- *Gratitude*: Writing a ten-item gratitude list nearly always counteracts almost any negative thought or mood.

- *Turn it over*: After recognizing a desire to control the behavior of another person (i.e., the addict), ask your Higher Power to take that desire away from you, and to please keep your addict safe.

Which stabilizing tools are you currently using regularly? Which of these tools works best for you?

_____

_____

_____

_____

_____

Do certain tools work better in certain situations? If so, which ones, and in what situations?

_____

_____

_____

_____

_____

What reasons do you give yourself for not using the tools you may need?

_____

_____

_____

_____

_____

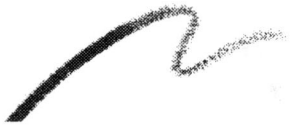

## Exercise 3
## Mindful Walking Meditation

The experience of an addictive crisis, is like being uprooted from the earth. At best, you will feel disconnected from your emotions. If the situation is especially bad, you could even have the feeling of "floating" or being dissociated from your body and your senses. These sensations are a traumatic stress response, and they are relatively normal when you experience the potential of losing connection to an addicted loved one, or when you sense that your own and your family's well-being is in jeopardy.

One way to combat these feelings is to engage in walking meditation. In all likelihood, you have engaged in various forms of walking meditation at some point in your life without even realizing it. Walking meditation is more than just strolling about. It is about being aware of your body and physical sensations as you move. Your eyes are open, and your mind and body are rooted in the current moment.

Benefits of walking meditation include the following:

- It can help you develop gratitude and understanding of difficult life situations.
- It gets your body moving and the blood circulating.
- It can assist in providing personal insight.
- It can easily be integrated into your schedule.
- It gives you an opportunity to remember and connect to the earth and nature.

To get started with walking meditation, take the following actions:

- *Pick a place.* Look for a place where you can walk slowly without obstacles. The location needs to be peaceful and devoid of traffic, and ideally it should be flat enough that you don't have to worry about stumbling. If you're walking in a public space, you'll need to take care not to get in the way of others. Practicing indoors may be a good option since you can focus directly on mindfulness with fewer opportunities to be distracted by your surroundings.
- *Get started.* After you've found a suitable place, begin each session by anchoring yourself. Take a minute to breathe deeply as you bring your full attention to your body. Sense how stable the ground feels beneath your feet. Be aware of the many different sensations within your body. Take

note of your thoughts and feelings as well. Now, start walking slowly. Rather than focusing on your breath, direct your attention to the movement of your feet and legs and the motion of your body as it advances. Just walk slowly and mindfully in a circle or back and forth. If you're turning around or turning a corner, be as mindful as you can of the position of your feet and the accompanying sensations. Do this for at least ten minutes. If necessary, take a break and stretch or simply stop moving and check in with yourself.

- *Maintain mindfulness as you walk.* As you observe the varying physical sensations that manifest as you walk, take note of your feelings, thoughts, and moods. There is no need to make a list, analyze, accept, or reject. Just notice these mental events as they arise and go back to the practice of walking. Try not to be rigid or mechanical while you walk. Simply walk naturally with good will and an open heart. Go with the flow.
- *Speed and posture.* The pace of walking meditation ranges from slow to extremely slow. You can let your hands and arms swing loosely by your sides, hold them behind your back, or clasp them in front of your body around the height of your diaphragm or navel. Your leg muscles should be relaxed as you walk, your movement natural and comfortable. Walk with poise, keeping your body upright, aligned, and dignified. It may be challenging at first, but with practice, you'll get the hang of it.

*For more information about Walking Meditation, visit Mindworks.org.*

The next time you feel emotionally or psychologically triggered, particularly regarding your addicted loved one, engage in Walking Meditation for at least ten minutes – longer if that is possible. Write a paragraph about that experience in the space provided.

_____
_____
_____
_____
_____

After utilizing walking meditation, does it feel like a useful tool to you? Why or why not?

_____
_____
_____
_____
_____

## Bonus Skill
## 5-4-3-2-1 Grounding

Sometimes you don't have time or the ability to go on a Walking Meditation. Maybe you're at work, or stuck in traffic, or having dinner with your mother-in-law. In such cases, other grounding techniques can be utilized. One of our favorites – because it is both effective and non-noticeable – is described next.

Whenever you are stressed, experiencing anxiety, or find yourself emotionally disconnecting, take a few moments to connect with your five senses. To do so, mentally list:

- Five things you SEE (a chair, a soda can, a cat, sunshine, a painting).
- Four things you HEAR (the A/C, traffic, birds chirping, a clock ticking).
- Three things you FEEL (the nubby fabric on my chair, tightness in my neck, the ground under my feet).
- Two things you SMELL (lemon air freshener, new leather).
- One thing you TASTE (coffee).

The best thing about this grounding technique, as previously mentioned, is that you can use it any time, any place, for any reason. The people around you won't even know you're doing it.

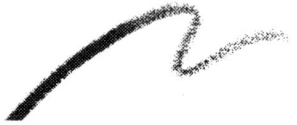

## Exercise 4
## Relaxation Breathing Exercises

Anxiety is the body's normal response to traumatic stress. It is a part of the fight/flight/freeze reaction that happens when you face a real or perceived physical or emotional threat. It can disrupt your everyday life and can become overwhelming. It can fill you with unease, distress, or dread.

We recommend breathing and related mindfulness exercises as a highly effective way for you to cope with anxiety associated with the addiction-driven relationship trauma you are going through. Such exercises can help you to slow your heart rate and feel calm.

We suggest that you practice each of the five techniques outlined next in times of stress. Pay attention to the benefits received from each technique. Note which practices work best in specific situations. Likely, you will find that some techniques are better with situational in-the-moment anxiety, while others are better with free-floating anxiety.

The best thing about breathing exercises is that they are easy and can be done almost anywhere, at any time. This means you can use them regularly throughout your healing journey for comfort, stabilization, relaxation, and calm.

The following five techniques listed are commonly used in meditation, therapy, and for coping with life in general. The instructions on how to utilize these techniques are adapted from an article by Amanda Barrell in *Medical News Today*.[1]

### Deep Breathing

1. Relax the stomach.
2. Place one hand just beneath the ribs.
3. Breathe in slowly and deeply through the nose, noticing the hand rise.
4. Breathe out through the mouth, noticing the hand fall.

### Quieting Response

1. Relax all the muscles in your face and shoulders and imagine having holes in the soles of your feet.
2. Take a deep breath, visualizing the breath as hot air entering your body through the holes in the soles of your feet.
3. Imagine the hot air flowing up your legs, through your tummy, and then filling your lungs.

4. Relax each muscle as the hot air passes it.
5. Breathe out slowly, imagining the air passing from your lungs back into your tummy, then your legs, before leaving your body through the holes in the soles of your feet.
6. Repeat until calm.

## Mindful Breathing

1. Sit or lie in a comfortable position with your eyes open or closed.
2. Inhale through your nose until your tummy expands.
3. Slowly let your breath out through your mouth.
4. Once settled into the pattern, focus on your breath coming in through the nose and out through the mouth.
5. Notice the rise and fall of your tummy as the breaths come in and out.
6. As thoughts come into your mind, notice that they are there without judging them. Then let them go and bring the attention back to your breathing.
7. Carry on until you feel calm. Then start to be aware of how the body and mind feel.

## Diaphragmatic Breathing

1. Start the process either sitting up or lying down.
2. Place one hand on your tummy and the other on the upper chest.
3. Breathe in through your nose, focusing on the tummy rising.
4. Breathe out through pursed lips, focusing on your tummy lowering.
5. Repeat the cycle.

## 4–7–8 Breathing

1. Sit down with your back straight up, your feet squarely on the floor, and the tip of your tongue on the back of your upper front teeth.
2. Breathe out through your mouth, making a whooshing sound.
3. Close your mouth and count to 4 while breathing in through your nose.
4. Count to 7 while holding your breath.
5. Count to 8 while breathing out through your mouth, making a whooshing sound.
6. Repeat at least three times.

Which of these exercises work best in reducing your situational, in-the moment distress?

_____

Describe the physical sensations when you use this technique.
*Example: I feel my shoulder muscles relax, and then the butterflies in my stomach go away.*

_____

_____

_____

_____

_____

Which of these exercises work best in reducing your free-floating, non-situational distress?

_____

Describe the physical sensations when you use this technique.
*Example: I feel the tension in my face relax, and then I feel sleepy.*

_____

_____

_____

_____

_____

Describe how you will make one or more of the breathing exercises previously described part of your regular routine?
*Example: I will add 4–7–8 breathing to my daily goals in the morning to help clear my head of stress, anxiety, and fears about the day.*

_____

_____

_____

_____

_____

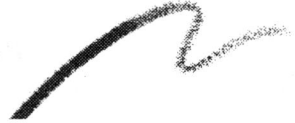

## Exercise 5
## The Self-Compassionate Eye

This exercise creates an adjustment to the way you may see yourself and messages you may say to yourself whenever you are in emotional pain. This pain is typically present when you feel sad, lonely, lost, betrayed, overwhelmed, afraid, rejected, unappreciated, etc. These new, more positive messages should speak to you individually. Thus, they can say whatever feels right to you. Here are some areas you may want to focus on.

- Identify and talk about the pain you are experiencing.
- Acknowledge the fact that pain is part of the human experience and that you are not alone.
- Decide to be kind to yourself in this painful moment.
- Write down a gentle message that will help you get through this painful experience.

The image is an example of a self-compassionate eye with self-compassion messages.

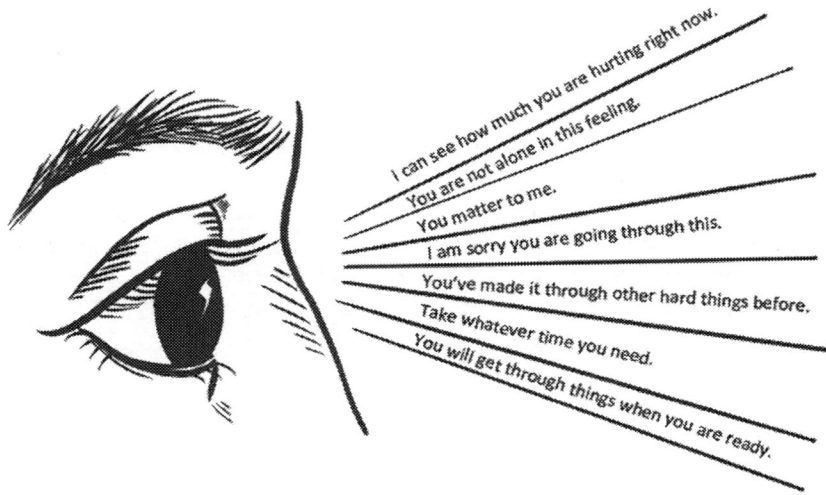

Based on the previous example, create your own self-compassionate messages.

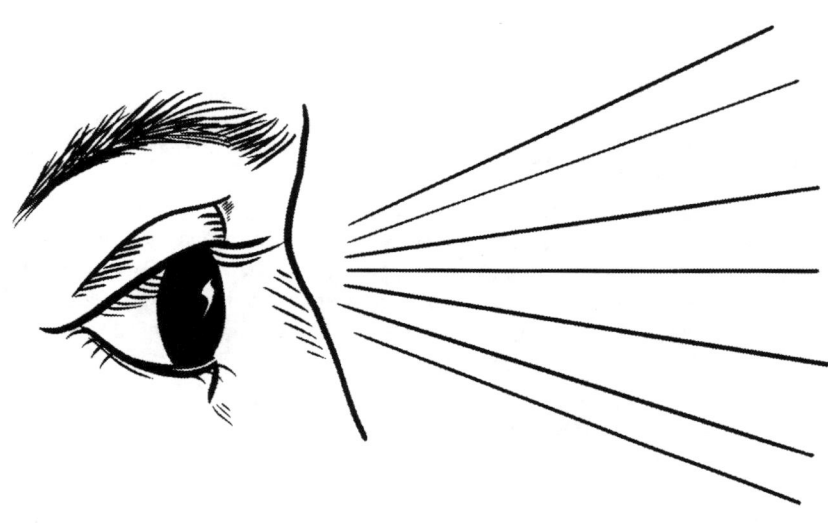

Explain how it felt to write these self-compassionate messages?
*Example: Writing these messages felt foreign and weird, but also good. It was a little confusing for me, but I didn't hate it.*

_____
_____
_____
_____
_____

Are you able to believe any of the messages from this exercise? What does that belief feel like?
*Example: I do believe that I am not the only one who has gone through what I am going through right now. Knowing that I am not alone makes me feel better, but it also feels bad that it happens to anyone.*

_____
_____
_____
_____
_____

Which of these messages do you reject today and why? Explain.

*Example: It is hard for me to believe that I can take whatever time I need to get through things. I feel like everything in my life is such a mess, I need to fix it NOW.*

_____

_____

_____

_____

_____

Explain what it might be like to give these messages to yourself in times of crisis and believe them?

*Example: It would feel good to be able to tell myself these messages, but I think it will take me a while to believe them.*

_____

_____

_____

_____

_____

Now take the self-compassion messages you created in this exercise and put them where you can see them and say them aloud at least two times per day (i.e., Post-it notes on your bathroom mirror). For the next week, do exactly that: State these self-compassion messages aloud at least twice per day.

After saying (and hearing) your self-compassion messages for an entire week, do you find it easier to take in these messages? To believe these messages? Explain.

_____

_____

_____

_____

_____

_____

_____

_____

_____

_____

_____

_____

_____

_____

_____

## Stage 2: Support and Connection

As stated, there are five primary goals of effective Prodependent treatment. The second of these involves the development of a support network and intimate emotional connections. Without question, a prevailing need for individuals experiencing relational difficulties caused by a loved one's addiction is to know that they are not the only ones who are going through the type of trauma they're experiencing. Challenging their shame and offering reassurance that their situation is not an isolated one is a key component of healing. The following four exercises are designed to be helpful in this regard.

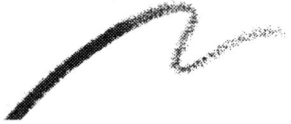

## Exercise 6
## Identifying Your Unmet Needs

As infants, all human beings have the three primary needs – food and water (sustenance), shelter, and emotional connection (love and stimulation). Infants are dependent on others for all three needs. Without the first two, they will die. Without the third, they become depressed, and often fail to develop and thrive.

These three basic needs do not go away as we grow older. We still need sustenance, shelter, and emotional connection as adults. And the consequences of going without are the same, including depression and a failure to thrive should our basic needs for emotional support are not met. Admittedly, this need looks different and is met in different ways during our adult years, but it does not disappear.

Examples of healthy adult emotional dependency needs are as follows:

- When I'm angry and I tell someone how angry I am, I want/need them to validate what I am feeling (to support, agree with, or at least acknowledge my anger).
- When I'm sad and I express my sadness to others, I want/need them to support, empathize with, and soothe me.
- When I'm joyous and I express this to others, I want/need them to validate, mirror, and cheer for me.

Emotionally healthy people naturally reach out to others – spouses, family members, longtime friends, lovers, therapists, clergy, support groups, and the like – when they have strong emotions, good or bad, that they need to regulate and process. Unfortunately, not every person is "emotionally healthy" in this way. And this lack of emotional health is especially likely when a person is in close relationship with an addict. In such cases, negative emotions and physical symptoms may cause an individual in crisis to sink deeper into despair.

Next is a list of dependency needs in four crucial areas: Physical, personal, relational, and spiritual. This list is neither exhaustive nor definitive. It is simply a starting point from which you can begin the process of identifying some of the unmet needs that drive your behavior.

As you examine this list, circle any needs that you feel *are not* being met. It is possible you will circle most or even all the items listed. If that happens, it is OK. Try to not judge yourself about what you have or have not identified. (An important thing you will notice as you complete the exercises in this workbook is that your needs will slowly and almost miraculously start to be satisfied.)

**Physical**: Things you need to care for your physical body and physical health.

Air
Food
Movement/exercise
Rest/sleep
Sexual expression
Safety
Shelter
Touch
Water
Protection
Clothing

**Personal**: Needs that address your feelings, growth, and what is most meaningful to you.

Honesty
Play
Autonomy
Creativity
Self-worth
Celebration
Challenge
Discovery
Contribution
Mourning
Choosing
Purpose
Understanding
Curiosity
Thought
Joy
Equality
Space
Spontaneity

**Relational**: Things you need to build secure and stable connections with loved ones and others.

Community
Inclusion
Intimacy
Belonging
Acceptance
Love

Respect
Companionship
Affection
Support
Compassion
Trust
Safety
Boundaries
Stability
Empathy

**Spiritual**: Needs that are connected to your intrinsic value and spiritual self – as you define it.

Harmony
Beauty
Peace
Inspiration
Order
Hope
Optimism
Forgiveness
Surrender
Guidance
Direction
Purpose

Of the unmet needs circled previously, pick three that seem most important to you. Note that each person has different needs, so there is no need to pick "the right three." Just pick the ones that stand out to you. In the space provided, explain how you would know if each of these needs was being met, and what you might do in the future to help that happen.

Example: Support. I would know I was being supported if I felt like my ideas and beliefs were being thoughtfully considered and given full weight. To feel supported, I will need to be more open about what I am thinking and feeling, especially with friends and family. I might even need to tell those people that I'm feeling vulnerable, and I really need them to "hear" what I'm saying.

Need 1: _____

_____
_____
_____
_____
_____
_____

Need 2: _____

_____
_____
_____
_____
_____
_____

Need 3: _____

_____
_____
_____
_____
_____
_____

List the three most important people in your life and write a sentence about how they do and do not meet your needs. Please note whether any of these individuals are addicted or struggling in some other significant way. Then ask: If they are not meeting your needs, do you think they are capable of doing so? If so, how might you facilitate that?

Example: My husband. Active addict. I do not feel that my husband meets my need to feel supported. I do, however, believe that he does love me and that he can give me what I need emotionally. To make this happen, I will need to tell him that I sometimes feel undervalued and underappreciated. When this happens, I will need to remind him of my emotional need to feel supported, asking him to "bring me in."

Person 1: _____

_____
_____
_____
_____

Person 2: _____

_____
_____
_____
_____

Person 3: _____

_____
_____
_____
_____

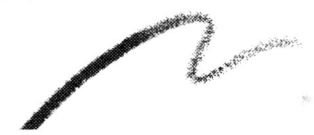

## Exercise 7
## Meeting Your Needs

Setting daily goals for getting your needs met can help you make that happen. These goals can also help you stay balanced as you experience the ups and downs of the healing process. If, for example, you notice that you are struggling more than usual, it is wise to check in on your goals to see how you are doing with them.

Sometimes, when life is difficult, it is easy to forget about your needs. This is doubly true when an addicted loved one is active in their addiction or struggling in their recovery. Recognizing this, we have created an exercise to help you identify, track, and meet your needs consistently. It is important that you not judge or shame yourself if you find that meeting your needs-related goals is difficult. Just do the best you can, and with practice and time, the process will get easier.

Set and track two daily goals in the following four areas:

- *Physical*: Things you need to care for your physical body and physical health.
- *Personal*: Needs that address your feelings, growth, and what is most meaningful to you.
- *Relational*: Things you need to build secure and stable connections with loved ones and others.
- *Spiritual*: Needs that are connected to your intrinsic value and spiritual self – as you define it.

We suggest that for the first few weeks you do this, you start with smaller goals that seem achievable and manageable. Over time, as you get better at setting and meeting your goals, you can move forward into larger needs-based goals. We also suggest that at least a few of your goals involve reaching out to other people, especially supportive, empathetic people who know about your process of healing.

## Sample Chart

Week of:   <u>March 14–20</u>

| *Area* | *Need Being Met* | *S* | *M* | *T* | *W* | *T* | *F* | *S* |
|---|---|---|---|---|---|---|---|---|
| Physical | Get at least 7 hours of sleep. | x | x | x | x | x | | |
| | Take a walk. | x | | x | x | x | | |
| Personal | Play the piano. | x | x | x | x | x | x | x |
| | Read a book for fun. | x | x | | | x | | |
| Relational | Text or call a friend. | x | x | | | x | x | |
| | Spend at least 10 minutes of one-on-one time with one of my kids. | x | x | x | x | x | | x |
| Spiritual | Meditate. | x | x | | | | | x |
| | Read something inspirational. | x | x | x | x | x | | x |

Now it is your turn. For the coming week (and hopefully beyond), create and track goals for yourself using this chart as a guide. You can make copies to use in future weeks.

Week of: _____

| Area | Need Being Met | S | M | T | W | T | F | S |
|------|----------------|---|---|---|---|---|---|---|
| Physical | | | | | | | | |
| Personal | | | | | | | | |
| Relational | | | | | | | | |
| Spiritual | | | | | | | | |

After setting and tracking your daily goals this past week, what did you learn about yourself?

_____
_____
_____
_____
_____
_____
_____

Did having stated goals and knowing you were tracking them help you meet the needs you identified?

_____
_____
_____
_____
_____
_____
_____

What does it feel like when your daily needs are met vs. when they are not met?

_____

_____

_____

_____

_____

_____

_____

_____

How do you feel this exercise affected you? For example, did you feel better about yourself, more overwhelmed, or more emotionally stable? Explain.

_____

_____

_____

_____

_____

_____

_____

_____

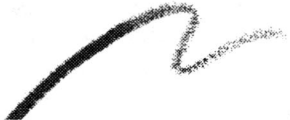

## Exercise 8
## List of Support

When you are dealing with an interpersonal crisis, it is crucial that you find support from someone other than the person who is creating the crisis (someone other than your addicted loved one).

To help yourself understand the support that is available (and not available) in your life, complete the following chart. Identify the names of those who are a general support to you, and those who are a healing support to you – meaning those who are available to help you through your current, addiction-driven difficulties.

| Category | General Support | Healing Support |
|---|---|---|
| Partner | | |
| Family | | |
| Friends | | |
| Support Community | | |
| Religious Community | | |
| Colleagues | | |
| Neighbors | | |
| Other | | |

Are there people listed in this chart who are currently providing general support who could provide healing support? If so, who, and what is their relationship to you? What characteristics do they have that suggests they could provide healing support?

*Example: My friend Susan. She is empathetic and her father was an alcoholic, so she understands the disease.*

1. _____

_____

_____

_____

_____

2. _____

_____

_____

_____

_____

_____

3. _____

_____

_____

_____

_____

How would you go about asking each of these individuals for healing support?

*Example: I have never really shared anything personal with Susan, but she has been a very loyal friend that I have not felt judged by. I think I will let her know some of what I am going through and find out how she responds.*

1. _____

_____

_____

_____

2. _____

_____

_____

_____

_____

3. _____

_____

_____

_____

_____

Are there people in your life who are not on this chart that you would like to be on it? If so, who, and what is their relationship to you? Why would you like these individuals to be on your chart?

*Example: John, my next-door neighbor. He is always friendly and kind to my entire family. He always says, "If you ever need anything, feel free to ask," and he seems to genuinely mean that.*

1 _____

_____

_____

_____

_____

2 _____

_____

_____

_____

3 _____

_____

_____

_____

How would you go about asking them for healing support?

*Example: John has confided in me about some of his own personal struggles. I would like to get to know him better and see if he would be someone who could be on my healing support list. I will start by inviting him to lunch so I can get to know him better, maybe sharing something about my story with him to see how he handles it.*

1 _____

_____

_____

2 _____

_____

_____

3 _____

_____

_____

Are there any people on this chart that you would like to remove from this chart? If so, who, and what is their relationship to you? Why would you like to remove them from your support network?

*Example: Andrew, my coworker. Andrew has not always kept my confidences, so I do not really trust him. I would like to keep him as a friend, but I no longer want him as one of my support individuals.*

1. _____

_____

_____

_____

_____

2. _____

_____

_____

_____

_____

3. _____

_____

_____

_____

_____

Do you feel like you are getting enough support from enough people, or do you need to continue to build your support network? Explain.

_____

_____

_____

_____

_____

_____

_____

_____

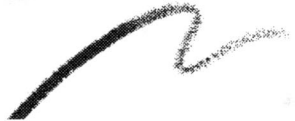

## Exercise 9
## Call to Courage

Facing relationship challenges can cause you to feel isolated, alone, and unsure of how to find connection and help from others. It will take courage for you to find a community and individuals who are trustworthy and willing show up for you when you are struggling. Many people, rather than ever reaching out for this kind of help, will simply assume rejection and not ask. From a healing perspective, this is debilitating.

To fully heal, you must take a few risks. One of those risks is becoming vulnerable and asking for help. This takes courage, especially when an important relationship (your connection with your addicted loved one) is a giant mess. That can make even the strongest of people at least a little bit timid.

The following questions are created to help you identify and embrace your courageous self so you can more fully participate in the healing process – by asking for help.

How do you define courage?
*Example: I define courage as doing something when I didn't think I could.*

---
---
---
---
---

Describe an action, as it relates to others, that you have previously taken or could take in the future that you would consider courageous?

*Example: Not long ago I was having an incredibly challenging day. I was feeling scared and angry about what was going on in my life. When a girlfriend called about something unrelated, she noticed I was upset. Instead of pretending I was OK, I shared with her how I was feeling. She took time to talk to me about it. I think that was me being courageous.*

---
---
---
---
---

_____
_____
_____
_____

Describe how it would it feel for you to reach out to someone and disclose what is going on in your life?

*Example: It would be really scary to talk to someone about what I am going through. I would worry that they would tell other people, and those people would judge me and my family.*

_____
_____
_____
_____
_____
_____
_____
_____
_____

Is it possible to be an independent and capable person yet still open up and get help from others when needed? Write your thoughts in the space provided.

*Example: I have always thought of myself as someone who can take care of himself, and I was taught as a kid that asking for help meant I was weak. It would be hard for me to do, but I will try to find someone to talk to about my situation.*

_____
_____
_____
_____
_____
_____
_____
_____
_____
_____

## Stage 3: Basic Education and Information

As stated previously, there are five primary goals of effective Prodependent treatment with loved ones of addicts. The third of these is to provide Basic Information and Education. Providing clear and concise information and education about the client's experience will help the client manage the extreme fear and hopelessness that may accompany it. The following five exercises are useful in this regard.

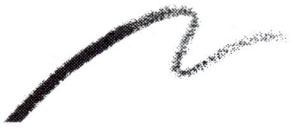

## Exercise 10
## Safety-Seeking Checklist

Sometimes, to create safety and protection after a relationship crisis, you will find yourself engaging in behaviors that are not necessarily helpful to you or your addicted loved one. Although your attempt to create safety is understand-able, the feelings experienced afterward are often shame, regret, pain, and confusion.

Whether your safety-seeking behaviors are healthy or not is for you to decide, as what is helpful and what is not helpful tends to vary from person to person. However, it is important that you can identify the safety-seeking behaviors in which you engage and that you recognize the ones that may be counterproductive and cause unnecessary stress and pain.

Next is a list of possible safety-seeking behaviors. Circle any behaviors that apply to you. The list we've provided is not exhaustive, so there is space to add some of your own.

Constantly checking on your struggling loved one.
Constantly checking in with your struggling loved one.
Looking through your struggling loved one's personal belongings for clues to their behavior.
Looking through phone records.
Checking the history on your struggling loved one's computer and phone.
Asking friends, associates, or colleagues questions about your struggling loved one.
Obsessing about where your struggling loved one is at any given moment.
Engaging in solicitous behaviors to connect with your struggling loved one or to control their behavior.
Talking about the trouble in your relationship with your struggling loved one whenever there is an opportunity.
Manipulating time, attention, and situations to try to control your struggling loved one.
Disclosing your struggling loved one's story to whomever you wish without their permission.
Using shaming and abusive language with your struggling loved one.
Other:
Other:
Other:

Explain which of the behaviors you circled seem to you to be counterproductive and therefore important to change, and why.

*Example: I secretly look through the computer history for evidence of my wife's infidelity. I feel terrible when I do this. I can't stop and it takes over my day.*

———————————————————————————————
———————————————————————————————
———————————————————————————————
———————————————————————————————
———————————————————————————————
———————————————————————————————
———————————————————————————————

Describe how you plan to accomplish this change (how you plan to stop your counterproductive behaviors)?

*Example: Rather than looking through the computer history for evidence of my wife's cheating, I will ask her to be open with me about her behavior. If I still feel that I need to see the online history, I will let her know about that, and I will stay within a specific time limit when doing it.*

———————————————————————————————
———————————————————————————————
———————————————————————————————
———————————————————————————————
———————————————————————————————

Are there any safety-seeking behaviors that you are engaging in that you did not list? If so, what are they, and why did you choose to not to list them?

*Example: I did not list the tracker I put on my husband's phone so I can see where he is at all times. I didn't list that because I am ashamed that I have to do that to feel safe.*

———————————————————————————————
———————————————————————————————
———————————————————————————————
———————————————————————————————
———————————————————————————————

Whom would you be willing to share your list with so you can ask for their help in changing your unproductive behaviors? Explain what this would be like for you.

*Example: I would be willing to share the list with my brother, but it won't be easy because I don't usually ask people for help.*

———————————————————————————————
———————————————————————————————
———————————————————————————————
———————————————————————————————
———————————————————————————————

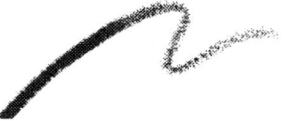

## Exercise 11
## Balance – the Rowboat

Learning to live life in balance is not easy, especially when you are living with the pain and stress of relationship/personal crises wrought by a loved one's addictive behavior. That said, creating balance for yourself is important to make the necessary changes that will bring you more peace and stability. You will feel out of balance when you do too much of any one thing. The first step toward achieving balance is identifying your stressors – the *waves of life* – so you can counter them with healthy and stabilizing behavior. You will also need to stay aware of warning or *threatening behaviors* that, when not acknowledged or adjusted, might take you back to old, unhelpful patterns.

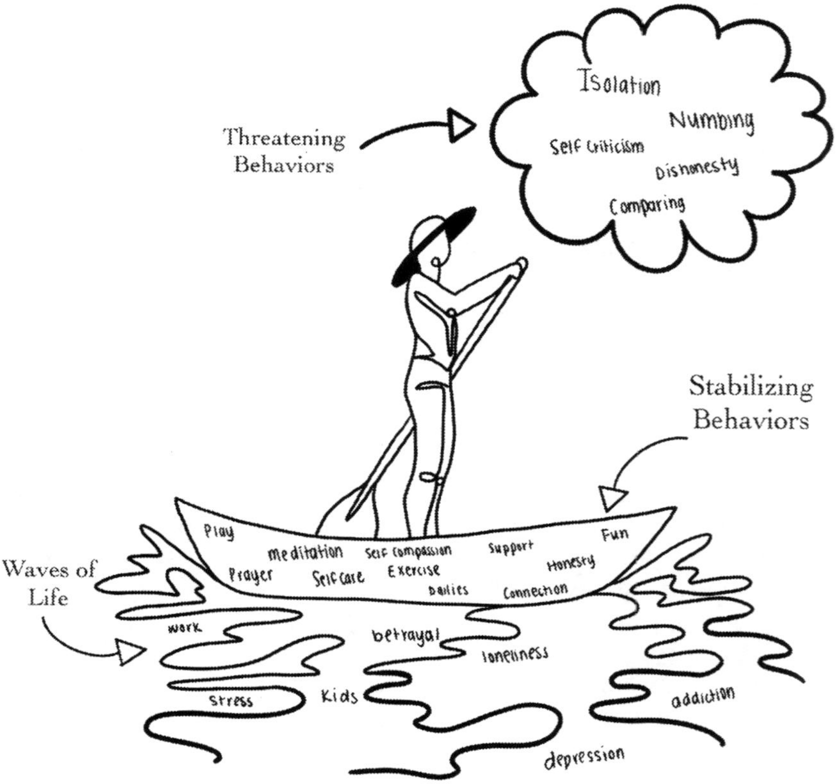

Threatening Behaviors

Isolation
Numbing
Self Criticism
Dishonesty
Comparing

Stabilizing Behaviors

Play
meditation   Self Compassion   Support   Fun
Prayer   Self Care   Exercise   Honesty
Dailies   Connection

Waves of Life

work
betrayal
loneliness
stress   Kids   addiction
depression

Counterbalancing life stressors with healthier *stabilizing behaviors* will help keep you steady in your "rowboat" when the waves of life happen.

On the next picture, identify and list your threatening and stabilizing behaviors, as well as the rolling waves of your life. You may want to complete this exercise using a pencil, as balance is something you will need to reevaluate and adjust as things change in your individual situation.

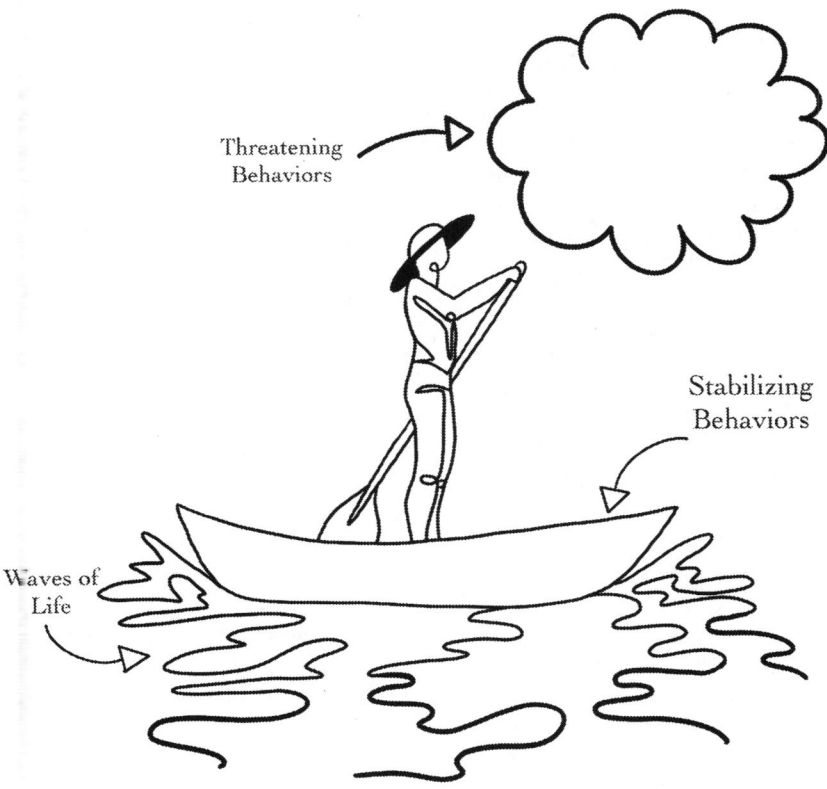

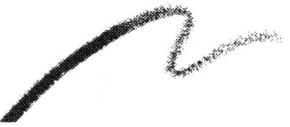

## Exercise 12
## Shame Prevention Plan

Brené Brown defines shame as the intensely painful feeling or experience of believing you are flawed and therefore unworthy of acceptance and belonging. She notes that shame creates feelings of fear, blame, and disconnect. Shame distorts your thoughts and feelings by telling you that something is wrong with you. It may tell you that you are not worth loving or nurturing and that you don't deserve to get your needs met in any relationship.

The Shame Prevention Plan described next is designed to help you identify shame and the ways in which it affects your life. It will aid in healing the negative beliefs that may have evolved over time about yourself and the world. Developing resilience to shame messages and being able to stabilize emotional distress requires you to challenge shame and turn negative internal messages and behaviors into healthier and productive coping strategies.

The Shame Prevention Plan can help you:

- Recognize when you are feeling fear and create tools to get out of it.
- Learn from the past and move into healthier patterns more quickly in the future.
- Reframe self-critical thoughts, turning them into new and more self-compassionate ones.
- Create awareness and ability to pursue healthier living and personal goals.

Shame Prevention Plans use specific terminology, described next.

*Activators*: Emotional, environmental, sensory, or situational stimuli that can elicit a trauma response linked to the distress you feel related to your addicted loved one. Activators can set in motion obsessive thoughts and fears. Exposure to activators is not your fault. Activators usually happen without warning and unsolicited. Either way, they can cause a lot of distress.

Examples:

- Seeing someone who looks like your spouse's affair partner.
- Watching a movie in which a bar scene is depicted.
- Looking through family albums and seeing happier times.

*Feelings*: Feelings are the emotional states that are set in motion when activators occur.

Examples:

- Sadness
- Anger
- Loneliness

*Shame-Based Beliefs*: These are the negative beliefs about yourself that are present when activators and the accompanying feelings occur.

Examples:

- Maybe something is wrong with me.
- Everyone else seems to be loveable. Maybe I'm just not.
- No one is there for me. I can't trust anyone in my life.

*Critical Thoughts*: These are the immediate thoughts that happen when shame-based beliefs are activated.

Examples:

- I'm such an idiot for marrying this person. I guess I'm getting what I deserve.
- My kid is probably going to end up in jail anyway. I don't know why I keep trying.
- If I hadn't been so mean, maybe they would still be sober. It's all my fault.

*Compassionate Thoughts*: With compassionate thoughts, you reframe your critical thoughts into healthier, more compassionate ones.

Examples:

- I married my partner because I felt like I should and because I believed in him. His choices after that do not reflect a problem with me.
- I keep trying because I love my kid and want more than anything for him to be healthy and happy.
- Even though I wish my interactions yesterday with my family members were healthier, the choice to relapse is not about me and is not my fault. I can only own what is mine.

Based on the information provided previously, work through a recent shameful situation. You may want to make a copy of this exercise to use in future situations.

## Shameful Situation:

*Example: I was talking to a friend, and she was telling me how close she and her husband are and how much fun they have together. I wanted to run away because all I could think about was how bad my relationship with my husband is and how many problems we have.*

_____

_____

_____

## Activators:

*Example: Listening to my friend gush over her relationship.*

_____

_____

_____

## Feelings:

*Example: I felt angry at my husband and at myself for being with him.*

_____

_____

_____

## Shame-Based Beliefs:

*Example: I can never count on my husband to be there for me.*

_____

_____

_____

## Critical Thought #1:

*Example: I am a loser for not being strong enough to leave him.*

_____

_____

_____

## Compassionate Thought #1:

*Example: Even though leaving seems like the easy solution, the truth is there are good things about our relationship.*

_____

_____

_____

**Critical Thought #2:**

_____
_____
_____

**Compassionate Thought #2:**

_____
_____
_____

**Critical Thought #3:**

_____
_____
_____

**Compassionate Thought #3:**

_____
_____
_____

Explain what it feels like to turn your critical thoughts into compassionate thoughts?

*Example: It is strange because the critical thoughts are so much easier to say (and believe) than the compassionate ones.*

_____
_____
_____
_____
_____

Explain what it feels like to stop blaming yourself for the addict's choices and behaviors?

*Example: I am so used to blaming and being hard on myself about my husband's choices. It is freeing to let go of that – even though it is hard.*

_____
_____
_____
_____
_____

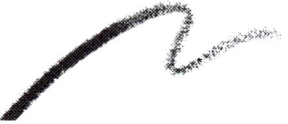

## Exercise 13
## Loss Inventory

Every person in relationship with an addict has experienced significant losses. Often, in the heat of the moment (as a caregiving loved one tries to keep the situation from blowing up), these losses are simply brushed to the side. In such cases, these losses may be forgotten (although they are never *really* forgotten) or ignored. Either way, they are not acknowledged and, as such, they cannot be grieved and processed. So, they linger as festering resentments, hiding in the back of your mind and eating at whatever remaining sense of connection you have with your addicted loved one.

To fully heal, you must identify these losses and bring them into the light of day. Otherwise, they will hide in the darkest recesses of your brain and poison your thoughts – not just your thoughts about the addict, but life in general. In the spaces provided, take an inventory of your losses and consequences related to your relationship with your struggling loved one. For each example of loss, list a related consequence.

| Loss | Consequence |
| --- | --- |
| I lost trust in my husband because of his drinking and cheating. | That loss of trust keeps me up at night, so I am losing sleep and not able to function as well during the day. |
|  |  |
|  |  |
|  |  |
|  |  |
|  |  |
|  |  |
|  |  |
|  |  |

After you complete this inventory, create a visual representation of your losses and consequences. You might create a timeline that depicts your story, a collage that shows what you feel like after these losses and consequences, or any other representation that feels right to you. You will need to find time, a safe space, and whatever tools you may need to represent these losses (i.e., paper, markers, pencils, glue, scissors, etc.).

Explain what it felt like to identify your losses and consequences.

_____
_____
_____
_____
_____
_____
_____
_____

Explain what it felt like to create a visual representation of your losses and consequences.

_____
_____
_____
_____
_____
_____
_____
_____

Is there anything you forgot or purposely left off your list of losses and consequences? If so, describe that loss and its related consequences in the space provided, and then explain why you did not initially include it.

_____
_____
_____
_____
_____
_____
_____
_____

In the space provided, list five other (nonaddiction-driven) losses you've experienced in your life. Rather than trying to list your five biggest or most challenging losses, simply list the first five that pop into your mind.

1. _____
_____
_____

2. _____

_____

_____

_____

3. _____

_____

_____

_____

_____

4. _____

_____

_____

_____

5. _____

_____

_____

_____

_____

Can you see any patterns or connections between your addiction and nonaddiction losses? If so, what are they?

_____

_____

_____

_____

_____

_____

_____

_____

_____

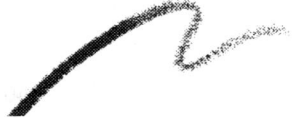

## Exercise 14
## Anger Inventory

When you are offended or betrayed by someone you love, this will usually pro-
voke feelings of anger. There are many ways that you may express this anger.
This exercise is designed to help you explore how your anger feels, how you
express it, and if you are avoiding it.

It is important that you understand that anger is a core emotion that is not
entirely negative. In fact, it can productively lead you toward taking needed
action. It can help you set and maintain boundaries and motivate you to take
steps toward change. That said, anger can also cause damage to yourself and
those you love if it is repressed or used as a weapon to punish yourself or hurt
another person. Thus, it is crucial that you learn how to feel and express your
anger appropriately.

It is common for loved ones of addicts to experience waves of anger that
come and go. Consider the moments of anger you've experienced since learning about your loved one's issues and problematic behaviors. Now, in the space
provided, list everything you've been angry about. Don't be afraid to list anything that comes to mind, and do not judge the anger you have felt.

*Example: I am angry that my son continues to lie and steal from me.*

1. _____

_____

_____

2. _____

_____

3. _____

_____

4. _____

_____

5. _____

_____

6. _____

_____

_____

7. _____

_____

_____

8. _____

_____

_____

9. _____

_____

_____

10. _____

_____

_____

Identify someone with whom you can share this list. Who is that person, and how does that person relate to your experiences with anger?

*Example: I can share this list with my brother. His son has done similar things and I don't think he will judge me or my son. He understands how addiction works because he is going through it too.*

_____

_____

_____

_____

_____

What does it feel like to have others identify with parts (or perhaps all) of the anger you have felt related to your struggling loved one? Explain.

*Example: It feels validating to know that I am not the only one who loves their kid but is also so angry with them for what they are putting me and the family through.*

_____

_____

_____

_____

_____

## Stage 4: Hope

As stated previously, there are five primary goals of effective Prodependent treatment. The fourth goal is to provide clients with Hope. Here, the therapist and client must strike a careful balance between providing and feeling some hope and managing expectations of future outcomes, particularly with the struggling loved one's recovery process. The following four exercises will be useful in this process.

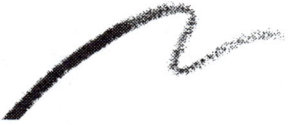

## Exercise 15
## The Grief Letter

Grief occurs when we have experienced significant losses in life and/or rela-tionships. According to Dr. Elisabeth Kübler-Ross, there are five stages of grief.[2] We have added an additional stage – remorse – as we believe it is an important and typical response for loved ones of addicts as they experience and work through (i.e., grieve) their relationship losses.

The stages of grief do not always follow one another sequentially. Moreover, they can repeat and/or cycle as grief is experienced and processed.

### Denial/Shock

- Disbelief that the disease, condition, or situation exists.
- No emotional acceptance.
- Sincere delusion, defensiveness.

### Anger/Defiance

- Hostile.
- If anger is not acceptable, feels guilty.
- Making others feel guilty, blaming.

### Bargaining

- Compromising, finding an easy way out, trying to *avoid pain.*
- Trying to keep "it" from happening.
- Trying to "run your own show."

### Depression

- Giving up. All is lost.
- No hope.
- Self-pity (Why me?).

### Remorse

- Self-blame.
- Feeling responsible.
- Questioning decisions (Did I do enough? Did I do too much?).

## Acceptance

- Acknowledgment and surrendering.
- Just dealing with "what is," not fighting or denying.
- Letting go.

Grief is never fun to experience. The upside of grief, however, is the final stage of the process: Acceptance. When grieving individuals reach acceptance, they can once again become hopeful about their lives.

Use the space provided to write about your grief. You might express feelings about what it is like to have grief present in your life, what you hope to learn from your grief, how you plan on overcoming your grief, etc.

_____
_____
_____
_____
_____
_____
_____
_____
_____
_____
_____
_____
_____
_____
_____
_____
_____
_____
_____
_____
_____
_____
_____
_____
_____
_____
_____
_____
_____
_____

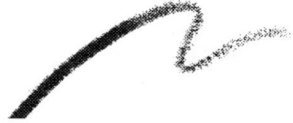

**Exercise 16**
**My Rights Manifesto**

Boundaries (which you will work on in Exercise 19) are meant to protect things of value. In this case, that thing of value is you! Before you can establish effective and appropriate boundaries, you will need to be able to clearly identify and embrace your own personal rights. Complete your list of personal rights in the next graphic.

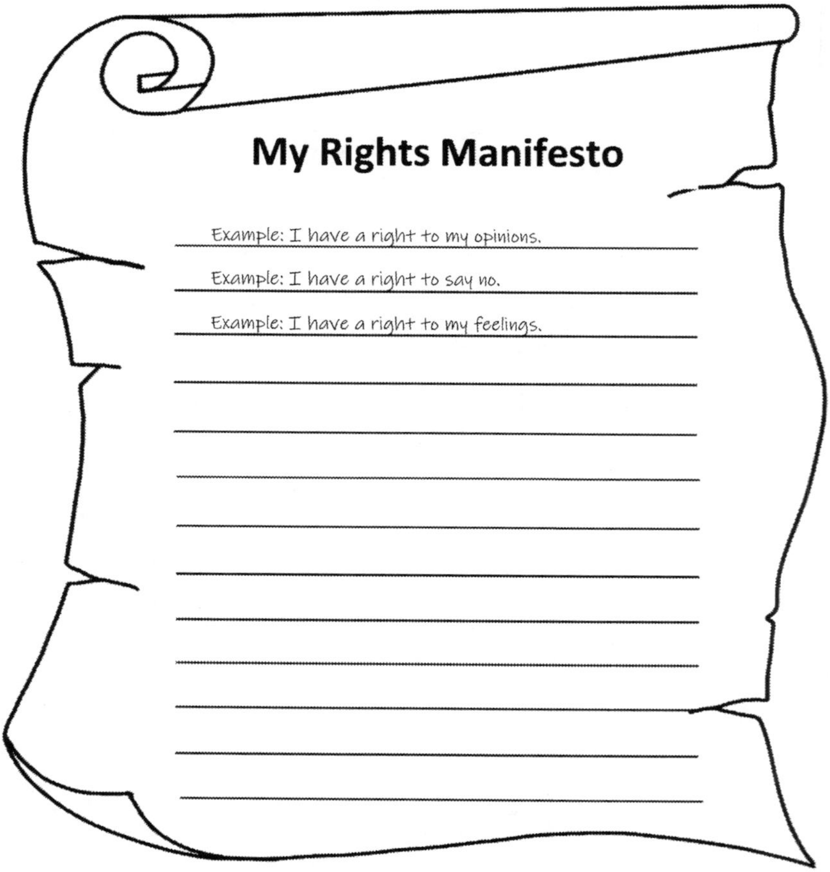

# My Rights Manifesto

Example: I have a right to my opinions.

Example: I have a right to say no.

Example: I have a right to my feelings.

Do any of the personal rights you listed not feel true? Why not?

*Example: I am not sure about being able to express my opinions. I want it to be true, but in my relationship, the addict almost always disagrees or thinks his opinion is right.*

_____
_____
_____
_____
_____
_____
_____
_____
_____
_____

Describe which of the personal rights that you listed feels the easiest to believe and why?

*Example: Even though my son doesn't think I should, sometimes for my own sanity, I have to say no.*

_____
_____
_____
_____
_____
_____
_____
_____
_____

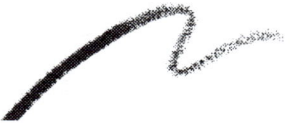

## Exercise 17
## Loving Support

Consider the "old ways" you have attempted to show love and to help your addicted loved one. Think about how some of your attempts have been ineffective or poorly received. List these unhelpful/unwelcome attempts at loving in the left-hand column. Then consider an alternative or Prodependent "new way" to provide love and support to the addict in that same situation. List that new way in the right-hand column.

As you complete this exercise, do not worry about getting it exactly right. The purpose of this exercise is not to come up with the perfect solution that will make everything OK in every situation; it is to bring to light the idea that some of what you've been doing is not working, and alternative behaviors may be available.

Consider the following examples.

| OLD WAY | NEW WAY |
| --- | --- |
| I help her schedule therapy appointments. | I can ask her to schedule her own appointments while letting her know that doing so will help me feel more secure. |
| I have him give his phone to me every night, so he won't be tempted to get on the Internet and look at pornography. | I can let him know I feel scared when he has his phone close to him all night, and I can ask him if he would be willing to do something different with it. |
| I know he cares about me or not if he plans and follows through with a fun date for us every Friday night. | I can let him know that going on a weekly date is important to me, and I can ask if we can alternate weeks planning it. |
| I installed a tracking app on her phone so I can see where she is at any time. | I will let her know that I feel afraid when I don't know where she is. Then I can ask her to be more transparent with me about where she is and what she is doing. |
| I frequently call or email his therapist and ask for updates about what he is accomplishing in therapy and how he is doing with his sobriety. | I will explain to him that having more information about his recovery helps me to feel safer and that it also helps to rebuild trust. |
| I reach out to his sponsor and let him know when he does things that do not look very "healthy" to me. | I can let him know when I see things in his behavior that concern me. |

Based on the previous examples, complete the following chart.

| OLD WAY | NEW WAY |
| --- | --- |
| | |

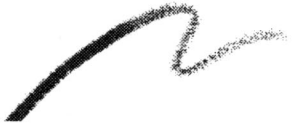

## Exercise 18
## Personal Serenity Mantra

*The Serenity Prayer*

Grant me the serenity to accept the things I cannot change,
The courage to change the things I can,
And the wisdom to know the difference.

Read the serenity prayer. Consider the words and what they mean to you. Consider how this prayer (or the meaning of the prayer) might help you in your ongoing process of letting go of the things you can't control.

Create your own unique serenity mantra or prayer.

*Example:*

May I learn to be kind to myself while I heal.
Learn to accept what has happened in my life.
And believe there is hope for brighter days ahead.

_____
_____
_____
_____
_____

Explain what it felt like to create your own serenity mantra/prayer.

_____
_____
_____
_____
_____
_____
_____
_____
_____
_____

## Stage 5: Healing

As stated previously, there are five primary goals of effective Prodependent treatment. The fifth of these goals is to facilitate Healing. For therapists, this means creating a generalized overview of the healing path ahead for both the client and the client's addicted loved one. This helps the client plan ahead. It also helps the client manage expectations and not be so disappointed as bumps in the journey naturally and inevitably arise. The following four exercises are designed to facilitate this process.

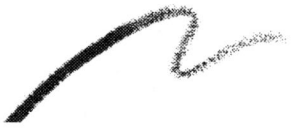

## Exercise 19
## Healthy Boundaries

Boundaries are limits established to keep yourself and others safe. Boundaries communicate respect for yourself and for the other person because they clarify the needs and wants of each individual. Learning to set and maintain effective boundaries is an important part of your healing process. Because relationships that involve an addiction or some other serious struggle often have damaged, ineffective, or nonexistent boundary systems, the need for healthy, effective boundaries is foundational to your healing.

Secure and stable attachments with others is not possible without boundaries that help to identify what is and what is not OK within the relationship. Having appropriate boundaries helps clear a path for authentic and steady connection. Boundaries are not established to push others away; instead, boundaries are set to bring others closer in a safe way.

There are six primary areas – or categories – of life that require boundaries:

- Physical: The ability to protect personal space, belongings, and your body as you see fit.
- Emotional: The ability to experience and express feelings and emotions openly.
- Relational: The ability to connect and nurture important relationships.
- Sexual: The ability to experience sexuality only as you feel comfortable.
- Thinking: The ability to have and express beliefs, reality, and understanding.
- Spiritual: The ability to express your understanding of what personal spirituality means.

The two basic types of boundaries are internal and external. Both types of boundaries provide safety in your relationship(s) as you navigate through the tumultuous waters of healing and reattachment.

- Internal boundaries are those that you establish for yourself. Generally, these need to be established and maintained before you will be able to create external boundaries.

  - Example: I will be honest with myself about what is happening in my life and the addict's life. I will no longer pretend that everything is OK when it clearly is not.

- External boundaries are those that you establish with others. Establishing healthy external boundaries will help you maintain the space you need to heal without completely detaching from your struggling loved one.

  ○ Example: When my husband is drinking and starts to become abusive, I will take the kids and go to my parents' house until he is sober.

## Basic Guidelines for Healthy Boundaries

- Boundaries are for personal safety and well-being, not for controlling others' behavior.
- Boundaries require consequences when violated; however, consequences should be steps the boundary setter will take rather than steps the boundary-crosser will take.
- Both individuals in any relationship should have clear boundaries.
- Boundaries are not barriers. Good boundaries simply communicate what is OK and what is not OK.
- Boundaries are fluid and need constant reconsideration and revision.
- Boundaries are not negotiable. They are about you; it doesn't matter if the other person likes or appreciates your boundaries.

## Boundary Setting

Think of situations you are currently experiencing where you would like to create more safety and security for yourself and others. As effective boundary setting might be new to you; we recommend that you start with smaller issues that feel more manageable and easier for you to maintain.

Examples:

| Boundary Type (Internal vs. External) | Category (Physical, Emotional, Relational, Sexual, Thinking, Spiritual) | Situation | Boundary | Consequence |
|---|---|---|---|---|
| Internal | Physical | Hugging my teenage kids without their permission. | I will ask them for permission before hugging them, and I won't guilt them if they say "no." | Quickly apologize and reestablish safety for them. |
| External | Relational and Physical | When my husband and I argue, sometimes he gets mad and leaves the house without telling me where he is going or when he will be home. I feel scared and unsafe when I don't know where he is. | "When you leave at night after we argue and don't let me know where you are, I feel scared, abandoned, and angry, I need you to let me know where you are, if you are safe, and when you plan to return." | "If you choose not to do this, I will need to go ahead and lock the house so I can sleep securely, and we can talk about it the next day, I will also feel more scared and disconnected from you, which could further damage our relationship." |

Practice creating your own boundaries. Try to list at least one boundary for each of the six categories – physical, emotional, relational, sexual, thinking, and spiritual.

| Boundary Type (Internal vs. External) | Category (Physical, Emotional, Relational, Sexual, Thinking, Spiritual) | Situation | Boundary | Consequence |
| --- | --- | --- | --- | --- |

Which of these boundaries are you ready to implement and follow through with right away, and which of these boundaries might need to wait until you feel stronger? What scares you about implementing the boundaries that need to wait?

_____

_____

_____

_____

_____

_____

_____

_____

_____

_____

_____

_____

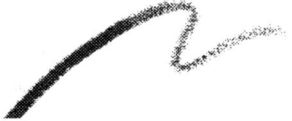

## Exercise 20
## Letting Go

Letting go is a concept that involves surrendering things that cannot be controlled. It is often painful when you realize that things you have attempted to control have actually caused you, and perhaps your addicted loved one, more pain and distress than relief. At the end of the day, all you can control is yourself. You cannot force others (especially addicts!) to change their thinking and behavior. You can set healthy boundaries around their behavior, but you cannot control their behavior. (Remember, healthy boundaries are about you, not the other person.)

Sometimes you have to just let others think as they think and do as they do, placing control in the "hands" of someone or something other than yourself. You may decide to turn things over to your Higher Power (however you conceive that entity), to the universe, or to anything else you deem powerful enough to hold and care for you and those around you. What's important here is your willingness to acknowledge what is and what is not in your power to control and change. Often, you will find yourself deliberately choosing peace over being justified or right.

### The Practice of Letting Go

Plan and engage in an activity that will represent how and what things you want to let go of. The following are some examples:

- Write down the things you would like to surrender on small pieces of paper and place them in some sort of container (often referred to as a *surrender box*).
- Write the things you are ready to surrender on paper and burn or shred each of them.
- Put small pieces of paper with what you are surrendering on them inside balloons. Then blow up the balloons with helium and release them into the sky.
- Write the items you are ready to surrender on rocks, put the rocks in a backpack, and hike with the backpack to a cliff or ledge. Then throw the rocks over the edge one at a time.

It is now time to create your own meaningful process. Start by making a list of ten things you are ready and willing to let go at this time.

*Example: The perfect fantasy I had about the future of my family and marriage.*

1. _____

_____

2. _____

_____

3. _____

_____

4. _____

_____

5. _____

_____

6. _____

_____

7. _____

_____

8. _____

_____

9. _____

_____

10. _____

_____

_____

Write out your plan for how you will surrender the ten things listed previously, and then carry that plan out with all ten items.

*Example: I will write down the specifics of the fantasy I had on a piece of paper, share it with someone I trust, and then burn it.*

1. _____

_____

2. _____

_____

3. _____

_____

_____

4. _____

_____

5. _____

_____

6. _____

_____

7. _____

_____

8. _____

_____

9. _____

_____

10. _____

_____

Explain what it was like to engage in this activity.
*Example: It felt a little silly and weird, but I did feel some relief.*

_____

_____

_____

_____

_____

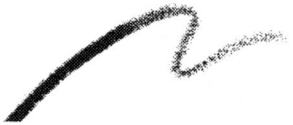

**Exercise 21**
**Reflection Artwork**

To honor all the difficult work you have completed to this point, use the space provided to draw a picture that represents your healing journey. Be sure to include where you have been, where you are currently, and where you imagine yourself going. Be sure to find time, a safe space, and whatever tools you need (markers, paper, pens, glue, photos, pencils, scissors, etc.) before you embark on this exercise.

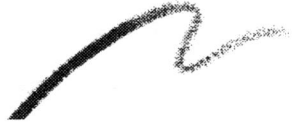

## Exercise 22
## Healthy Living Plan

The Healthy Living Plan outlines your intention to identify and establish healthy living patterns and routines.
Example of a Healthy Living Plan.

Healthy behaviors I will engage in:

* Creating a daily routine for self-care and meeting my dependency needs.
* Maintaining a support network.
* Seeking help from a mental health professional as needed.

How I will seek support: I will see my therapist at least once per week.

How I will exercise:

* I will exercise by going to the gym or hiking at least three times per week.

How I will eat:

* I will focus on eating three meals per day, with only healthy snacks in between.

How I will sleep:

* I will make sure to get at least six hours of sleep every night.

How I will take breaks:

* I will make sure to take a lunch break at work.

When I need support, I will call:

* My support group members.
* My brother.
* My coworker.

In the space provided, create your Healthy Living Plan.

Healthy behaviors I will engage in (refer to stabilizing tools):

_____

_____

_____

_____

_____

How I will seek support: _____

How I will exercise: _____

How I will eat: _____

How I will sleep: _____

How I will take breaks: _____

When I need support, I will call:

_____

_____

_____

_____

## Notes

1. Barrell, A., (2020). Five breathing exercises for anxiety and how to do them. *Medical News Today*. www.medicalnewstoday.com/articles/breathing-exercises-for-anxiety
2. Kübler-Ross, E., & Kessler, D. (2005). *On grief and grieving: Finding the meaning of grief through the five stages of loss*. Simon & Schuster.

# Section 5
# Prodependence FAQs

**Q: What are potential clinical roadblocks when moving from Codepend-ence-based to Prodependence-based treatment?**

A: One roadblock may be the clients are already well versed in Codependent language and history. They may have already been told they are Code-pendent and have been attending support meetings, read various books, and received Codependence-based counseling services. These clients may be more resistant to looking through a new lens in their healing. It may take time to help them acclimate to a new paradigm. Another challenge may occur when the treating therapist experiences difficulties adopting this new therapeutic language and viewpoint as there have been no other perspectives for many decades.

**Q: How does the 12-step recovery model fit into treatment if a loved one's safety-seeking behavior is no longer seen in terms of Codependent pathology?**

A: The 12-step recovery and support model can easily be modified to fit the Prodependent paradigm. In fact, proponents of this new concept have already started a new worldwide healing community called Prodependence Anonymous (www.Prodependenceanonymous.org). For those without the resources to attend therapy or related support groups, we highly recommend considering this kind of supportive, non-judgmental experiences.

The 12 steps of Prodependence Anonymous:

1. We admitted we were powerless over our attempts to heal those we love – that our lives had become unmanageable.
2. We came to believe that a power greater than ourselves could restore us to sanity.
3. We decided to turn our will and our lives over to the care of God *as we understand God.*
4. We made a searching and fearless moral inventory of ourselves.
5. We admitted to God, to ourselves, and to another human being the exact nature of how our actions have harmed ourselves and others.
6. We were entirely ready to have God remove our self-defeating actions and beliefs.

7. We humbly asked God to remove our self-defeating actions and beliefs.
8. We made a list of all persons we had harmed and became willing to make amends to them all.
9. We made direct amends to such people wherever possible, except when to do so would injure them or others.
10. We continued to take personal inventory and when we were wrong promptly admitted it.
11. We sought through prayer and meditation to improve our conscious contact with God, as we understand God, praying only for knowledge of God's will for us and the power to carry that out.
12. Having had a spiritual awakening as the result of these steps, we tried to carry this message to others and to practice these principles in all our affairs.

**Q: What defines Prodependence versus Codependence?**

A: The primary difference between Prodependence and Codependence lies in how we frame and think about "the problem." Prodependence recognizes that loved ones of active addicts are perpetually in crisis mode. Naturally, they try to control the crisis. In the process, they sometimes panic and make bad decisions. They may overdo. They may help too much. They may help ineffectively. They may regress by acting in ways that reflect their own early trauma; they may enable and appear to be pathologically enmeshed. But unlike Codependence, Prodependence *does not ascribe any pathology* to their actions (or thoughts). We do not view loving people in these types of situations as psychologically disordered as does Codependence. Prodependence views such people as amid a profound life crisis not of their own making. Thus, they are behaving in the ways that people in crisis tend to behave. Rather than blaming and labeling these loving people or asking them to explore themselves, Prodependence meets them where they are, which is coming from a place of understandable fear, anger, confusion, love, and a desire for attachment.

**Q: When is it appropriate to move into clinical work surrounding the loved ones' historical trauma history not related to their current crisis?**

A: As the Prodependence model is heavily focused on and influenced by crisis intervention work, the model is most applicable in the earliest stages of treatment while there is an ongoing crisis (the addict is not sober but the loved ones remain deeply invested in the relationship). When the client is out of the immediate crisis, including their confusing, dysregulating trauma symptoms, and we are seeing both emotional and physiological stabilization, then – should there be interest or a desire to do so by the client – we may begin therapies designed to assist and resolve historical issues. This is not to say that such clients don't have "trauma work" of their own to do. *However, we do not initiate introspective psychotherapy while our clients are managing the active or early stages of a meaningful life crisis nor do we seek to create to form a formalized, long-term diagnosis or treatment plan. This said, we must always intervene if clients are demonstrating active signs of being abused, engaging in self-abuse, acting out their own addictions or struggling with their own mental or physical health.*

Q: Can a client complete the workbook exercises alone, or do they need to be completed with an individual therapist or in group therapy?

A  The exercises are designed for use within a group (or individual) therapy setting with a professional mental health provider who has training and experience. However, they would also be useful to a facilitated or non-facilitated peer support group. There is not a prescribed length of time or structured lesson plan associated with their use, as that would be at the discretion of the clinician or individuals based on the specific needs of that individual or group. These basic exercises are intended to be a starting point for physiological, emotional, and behavioral stabilization. If any specific assignment might lead to emotional dysregulation, we simply pick another one or take time out from such assignments until the client is more stable.

Q: Prodependence is a 180-degree turn away from Codependence. What was so wrong with that model?

A: *Research Validity.* Codependence *is not and has never been a clinical diagnosis* – period. It has only ever existed as a pop-culture idea that was integrated into clinical literature. There is no valid past or recent research on the topic as none has been carried out since 1994! There are no universal diagnostic criteria available to determine if someone is or is not Codependent. It has never been in the DSM or ICD as a formalized diagnosis. There is not – nor has there ever been – a universal standard for what defines Codependency or how to treat it.

B: *One-Size-Fits-All Treatment.* It is not ethical to create an *automatic diagnosis* or label that is to be applied to anyone based on their circumstances. It is not ethical for professionals to apply labels or pathologies to any client when that client is in a crisis – as does Codependency. Further, it not ethical for professionals to apply labels or pathologies to any client that are not proven by scientific data. We wrote this book because decades of shared clinical experience have exposed us to far too many loving family members, friends, and spouses who addicts turned away from the help they so desperately needed because they felt judged by the very model being employed to treat them.

C: *Ineffective and Judgmental Treatment.* We have watched people who have literally exhausted themselves trying to save a loved one from addiction. People become angry, disappointed, and confused in their own therapy, feeling themselves to be blamed, misunderstood, and shamed by being labeled as Codependent. These same patients and clients tell us that Codependence felt like a label that was hung around their neck simply because they had an active addict in their life and/or because they are deeply caregiving by nature. While therapists have been busily pathologizing supportive families and loved ones of addicts as Codependent for decades, their chronically addicted partner, parent, or child is failing at school, getting fired from another job, or was recently arrested.

  *Professional Deficits*: We have seen many informed and compassionate and therapists lacking simple, useful answers to help such family members and caregivers. Such professionals have only one method to treat these people. Thus, they have been forced to rely on Codependence, a model that most often feels more negative and alienating than invitational. Prodependence provides another clinical option, one that recognizes the inherent grace of these caregivers, while applauding and validating their unconditional commitment, courage, and conviction to restore love and family.

*Cultural Bias:* Of primary concern is the fact that Codependency is near solely centered on Eurocentric beliefs that a crisis like addiction offers the individual an opportunity to differentiate and self-actualize. Most cultures do not view individualization, self-actualization, and detachment as the road to healing a crisis (like active addiction). Codependency is culturally biased as its foundational theories and goals are simply not applicable to cultures that place a higher value on community support than self-development.

*Gender Bias:* Codependency at its core stresses independence, self-actualization, and personal growth over interdependency. Codependent theory is sourced in foundational 20th century feminist beliefs that stressed independence and detachment over interdependence and shared relational dependencies. Women were then told that the road to success and achievement in a man's world required them to eschew their traditionally valued strengths of empathy, compassion, and community building. They were strongly encouraged to trade in these emotional traits and replace them with traditionally valued male strengths of competitiveness, assertion, and "going it alone." In this way Codependency overshot the mark by devaluing our very human, healthy need to lean into and gain support from those around us. Codependency encouraged women to become more anti-dependent than interdependent. These ideas, though useful at the time, are antithetical to current attachment theory, which is focused on the importance of healthy human dependency.

### Q: What is the major difference between Codependence and Prodependence?

A: *Codependence* is a model of human behavior sourced in the exploration of a client's *trauma history that states that those who partner with an addict or are responding to the desperate needs of an addicted family member are troubled by implication.* To "be Codependent" implies that one tends to bond deeply with those whose lives tend to mirror the early traumatic failures/traumas of their early childhood development. Failure on the part of the active addict then serves as a trigger for the nonaddicted partner to act out their unmet needs or abuse from childhood within this troubled adult relationship. Codependence implies that the loved ones of addicts, due to their underlying, often unconscious "childhood issues" tend to, as adults, give too much and love too much. Thus, they attract, enable, and enmesh with addicted partners. The goals of Codependency treatment revolve around themes of detachment, self-actualization, becoming less needy, and working through past trauma to become more aware, less enabling, and less accepting of troubled, emotionally unavailable people. Codependency is a deficit- and trauma-based model.

*Prodependence* is a model of human behavior based on *attachment theory.* To "be Prodependent" implies that one can create deep, bonded adult attachments that mirror our very human, normative longings for healthy dependence and intimacy. Prodependence assumes that, when one loves and bonds deeply, it is natural and therefore non-pathological to do whatever it takes to ensure the safety and stability of those with whom one is attached. Prodependence implies that loved ones of addicts, regardless of prior history, will take extraordinary measures to keep those they love stable and to ensure the safety of their families. There is no pathology assigned to loving in Prodependence. Rather, Prodependence asserts that loving addicts or other chronically troubled people healthfully requires a different form of love than that with healthy adults. Loving Prodependently requires support, guidance, and informed help. Prodependence is a strength-based, attachment-based model.

**Q: When did Codependence evolve into theory and practice?**

A: Codependence was initially promoted in six books published between 1981 and 1989, almost solely written by female therapists who worked in the addiction field. It meshed with and ultimately subsumed the preexisting co-addiction movement. Later, it broadened in the larger culture to include caregivers of all stripes, not just caregivers of addicts.

**Q: Why did Codependence become so popular?**

A: Codependence was an easy-to-understand, engaging concept, and it mirrored the culture of the era of its creation related to feminism, systems theory, and the human-potential movement of the 1960s–2000. These concepts are detailed in the original concept book *Prodependence: Ending the Myth of Codependency* but can also be found here in Chapters 2 and 3.

**Q: Can Codependence treatment be counterproductive when working with loved ones of addicts?**

A: Yes, and it frequently is. Codependence, by definition, implies that there is something wrong with the person who loves, rescues, helps, and cares for an addict. This is especially true if that person has given up essential parts of themselves in the process. Embracing the Codependence model requires convincing loving family members and friends, already amid a profound life crisis, that *there is something deeply wrong with them, that they are somehow encouraging the addiction* that they need to fix. As a result, increasing numbers of people now leave treatment before they receive the help they need and/or never reach out for such help.

**Q: If someone can be called Codependent, does that mean that someone can also be called Prodependent? What are the signs of being a Prodependent person?**

A: Prodependence is not a label or a diagnosis. No one is Prodependent. The term is meant to emphasize our healthy need to depend on other safe and supportive people in good times and in bad. It is meant to validate and define interdependent relationships where one naturally gives of oneself to a troubled other as healthy rather than pathological. The word Prodependence can be seen as a synonym for the concept of interdependence as applied to the families and loved ones of addicts in crisis.

**Q: Is this book suggesting that Codependency doesn't exist?**

A: Yes. When discussing problems of human dependency, the authors wish to strongly point out that long before the concept of Codependency was created, there were (and remain) far more descriptive, accurate, and validated terminology to describe such problems than the word Codependence. Formal clinical terms like *overdependence, unhealthy dependency, dependent personality disorder, along with the well-understood attachment (dependency) styles of secure, anxious, avoidant, and disorganized forms* are more useful as they are far more accurate.

Prodependence, as a concept and in practice, does not support the concept of Codependence. Prodependence sees Codependence as a theory that does not fully encompass the lived experience of addicts' loved ones, nor consider the needs of the situations they face with an active addict. Execution of the Codependence model in treatment tends to alienate the people it was designed to help, as it leaves them feeling more judged than supported. Additionally, the theory of Codependence has never been formalized as a clinical diagnosis. In fact, it was proposed and rejected by the American Psychological Association (APA) in the early 1990s.

**Q: How does Prodependence view the problem behaviors created by an addict's loved ones, such as enabling, overzealously caretaking, and even raging at the addict?**

A: Prodependence views all such activity as the caregiver's "best attempt" to save a troubled loved one. It sees these behaviors as loving – though sometimes less than ideal – efforts to save a person they care for. That said, Prodependence does not label or judge loved one who are sincerely trying to help the addict, whether or not their attempts were effective. Instead, Prodependence views these actions as a loved one's best effort to stay connected and help in a situation that they did not cause and that is beyond their ability to remedy. After all, most folks were not educated in high school or college on how to live with an addict or get them sober. So why would we expect them to know *the right ways to help* should someone they love become addicted?

**Q: How does Prodependence tackle typical challenges to treating loved ones of addicts, including emotional reactivity and enabling?**

A: As stated earlier, Prodependence rightfully acknowledges the fact that spouses, family, and friends of active addicts, no matter how caring, most often lack the specialized training or education that would equip them to help an out-of-control addicted person. It also recognizes the immense pain and fear that come along with witnessing a beloved person fail. Thus, it is perfectly understandable, when seen through a Prodependent lens, that such individuals will compensate for their lack of expertise with passionate, if at times misguided, attempts to help arrest the addictive process, thus leaving some of such attempts counterproductive. Prodependence does not ask the therapist to pathologize family members' attempts to heal someone they love as their feelings and actions are not regarded as arising out of anything but love. The goal is to support family members by validating their love while simultaneously helping them to develop the patience and skills to make their actions and words more effective and useful.

**Q: Does Prodependence say that there is nothing wrong with the loved ones of an addict, even when they exhibit problematic traits?**

A: Prodependence implies that such loved ones of addicts are caught up in circumstances that would naturally overwhelm anyone of us. Thus, there is nothing "wrong" with them, regardless of their personal history. They are trying as best they can to survive and to help their family survive extraordinary, overwhelming circumstances. What these caregivers require from day one is validation for the love and care they have given, direction for helping their troubled family member in healthier ways, and hope.

**Q: What about trauma? Don't many spouses of addicts have early childhood trauma?**

A: Yes, many spouses of addicts, much like addicts themselves, have had early or later-life traumatic experiences. In fact, these similar histories, both conscious and unconscious, are frequently part of what has bonded these people to one another. All of us may regress into acting out elements of past trauma when surviving the acute challenges presented by an actively addicted loved one. This is unsurprising, considering the extremely stressful and overwhelming circumstances addictions produce. That said, not everyone is suffering from the effects of early trauma. Either way, initial Prodependence therapy and treatment for families and loved ones of addicts does not seek to explore such issues. Instead, the therapeutic intention is to help and support these people by working toward self-regulation and crisis management.

**Q: How does Prodependence view and treat past trauma in partners of addicts?**

A: Prodependence sees an addict's partner as being in crisis when beginning treatment. Therefore, the treatment is initially intended to help this individual resolve their immediate crisis. After the crisis has been addressed, the client is encouraged to examine their personal history with the therapist, *should they display an interest*. However, Prodependence does not bind the reactions of someone living with an active addict to their past. Asking a partner to address trauma – or even to examine their own history – early in the recovery process can be abusive, as doing so implies an innate fault with the caregiver. Thus, this is not a priority early in the partner's treatment.

**Q: What happens when such loved ones are themselves emotionally disabled as to be actively interfering with the process of addiction healing?**

A: When loved ones are unable to be soothed, supported, or redirected in early treatment, this simply implies that they need care that is separate and apart from their immediate circumstances. Most frequently, they express familiar and readily diagnosable conditions like depression, anxiety, and/or reactivity to past traumatic events. As these individuals heal, their treatment can then be integrated into overall addiction family care.

**Q: What about the apparent need of "Codependent" people, in general, to self-actualize and grow, independent of their relationships and bonds?**

A: Prodependence, coming from an attachment-based perspective, says that all of us are deeply dependent on one another for emotional survival and that this is a good thing. Mutual, deep, and enduring dependencies from womb to tomb is how humans survive and thrive; as such, even troubled relationships should never be regarded as inherently pathological. Prodependence celebrates rather than pathologizes deep emotional dependency. It regards healthy, deeply bonded relationships of all kinds as key to an individual's self-actualization. Enmeshment is viewed merely as a misguided attempt to reengage a secure attachment that can be improved and redacted to become more successful.

**Q: Since Prodependence is filled with themes of partnership, attachment, and working toward connection, under what circumstances could a partner, family member, or loved one choose to leave the relationship with the addict – for a while or forever?**

A: The authors do not believe that anyone should remain in a situation that is painfully taking away their own sense of self and stability. Prodependence (unlike Codependency) is not a one-size-fits-all solution, nor is it meant to apply the same actions/philosophies for every situation. Our first job with clients should always focus on "safety first," defined on a case-by-case basis. Sometimes, the most loving and caring thing a client can do is leave – not to manipulate the addict – but rather in the service of their own safety and sanity. Maintaining loving connections and the hope for healing is near always possible but living with the problem in real time may not be

**Q: Is it OK to leave or ask the addict to leave out of frustration and sadness about the lack of change?**

A: No matter how much love clients have in their hearts, no matter the past history of good and bad times, sometimes there is no way forward. All the love and frustration and sadness cannot make the addicts change their behavior. That is up to them. The addicts may need the loved one – but sometimes they need the loved one to leave so they may struggle with their demons alone before getting help. The hardest of these client situations is when loved ones are holding onto caring and compassion for the addict but don't fully see how it is affecting their own mental, physical, relational, and emotional health first. There is no loving or helping another, especially a troubled other – without first having a personal foundation of stability. To leave doesn't necessarily mean the loved one has to leave forever, and it certainly doesn't have to mean ending the relationship (even though it may change form, say from a marriage to a friendship or co-parenting), but it does mean that the loved one's sanity and peace of mind must also be a priority.

**Q: Why leave if there is no overt abuse (hitting, violence, meaningful threats, etc.)?**

A: The damage inflicted on the individuals and the relationship where abuse is present, whether overt or covert, is the same. It may be difficult for the loved ones to understand why they feel so conflicted about leaving if the said "damage" is not obvious. We can help by providing education and understanding about the abuse and its impact on the loved ones, as well as assist them in figuring out the safest path moving forward.

**Q: What if the clients are simply done, how can they leave out of love or with love?**

A: Ending a troubled relationship in a respectful way is the responsibility of both parties. The therapist should first make sure the loved one is not in a current crisis where they are making the decision in a reactionary or trauma state. Once that stabilization is achieved (if necessary), the therapist can then gently break down the steps of moving forward with a step-by-step plan for exiting the relationship, while consistently assessing for as many factors as possible, including the client's stability and safety throughout the process.

**Q: What if the loved one is still deeply in love with the addict and wants a healthier relationship, but the addict remains emotionally unavailable because they are still using, lying, disconnected, etc.?**

A: Prodependence would celebrate the loved one's desire for connection and to build a healthy relationship; however, active addiction will make this practically impossible. The therapist will validate this desire, while simultaneously holding space as the loved one decides how long they will be able to wait for the addict to get sober and do the hard work of showing up in the relationship. The therapist will also remind the loved one that this change in the addict is not something they can control but rather hope for and do the best they can to take care of themselves in the meantime.

**Q:How do the loved ones deal with the anger/sadness/guilt inducing/ gaslighting/false promises of the addict after they decide to leave the relationship?**

A: Helping the loved ones create safety for themselves and other family members if necessary will be an important task for the treating therapist. When someone decides to end a relationship, particularly with someone who is not stable or in an active addiction cycle, anger and emotional lashing out are to be expected. Helping the loved ones establish guidelines and limitations for interpersonal interactions with the addict will be necessary to maintaining safety and security for everyone.

**Q:How do I help loved ones who are ready to leave the relationship but feel a lot of guilt and fear because the addict is still using?**

A: The therapist can reassure the loved ones that it is not their fault or responsibility to save or fix the addict, but it is understandable that they would experience internal conflict about their decision as they have spent a lot of time caring about and trying to help them. It might also be helpful for the therapist to help the loved ones identify and reach out to others who love and care for the addict to let them know of their decision and ask them to step in and help the addict where they can, effectively passing some of the heavy responsibility they have been carrying to others.

**Q:How do I help loved ones who feel guilty leaving the relationship even though the addict is sober?**

A: A Prodependent-based therapist would want to affirm the clients' decision to leave, being sure to help them understand and process their grief due to the out-of-control losses they have experienced in the relationship that led them to their choice. The therapist can also reassure the loved ones that grief has a beginning and an end, and it is OK if they are unable to continue in the relationship no matter the sobriety status of the addict.

**Q:What if the client cannot leave due to financial or childcare issues?**

A: Financial dependency can be a significant consideration when an addict's loved ones are deciding whether to stay in the relationship. It is not uncommon for a loved one to have spent their time in the relationship taking care of the home and children and not being the primary breadwinner. It is also not uncommon for the loved one to have a job but not make enough to support themselves. The therapist would have the role of assisting the loved one in finding and/or securing the resources to become self-reliant. This may take time and may delay the decision to leave, but it would be time well spent. The exception to this type of assistance would be if there is an immediate need to leave due to safety issues. In this case, the therapist would assist the client in finding resources that can provide protection and support until the loved one can be on their own. This may be the right time to see an attorney or other professional if possible to ensure that any finances are secure and not manipulated as a form of abuse.

**Q: What if there is abuse, does Prodependence suggest that the best way to work through this is by staying with the abuser?**

A: There is no situation where Prodepenence would encourage someone who is being physically or sexually abused (or their children) to remain around for more. We also understand that many addictive relationships will involve some degree of verbal abuse and psychological violation. Whether to stay or leave in such situations is best done case by case. It is always recommended for anyone who feels a lack of safety in their own home (or in the homes of those they love) to seek help, advice, direction, and interventions by experts in domestic violence as well as therapists trained to help in these circumstances.

**Q: How can the therapist best help a loved one weigh all the outcomes of their decision to leave?**

A: If the client has decided to leave an addictive relationship, one of our clinical tasks is to assist them in identifying and being clear about all possible consequences and scenarios surrounding that choice. This way, the client is less likely to find themselves in a situation that has not been previously considered, thereby getting a better chance of successfully navigating it. There is always the potential that the outcomes of leaving may not look or sound any better than staying and that either choice will come with its own set of challenges. However, planning the best they can for these outcomes can bring peace and some semblance of control over their own reality – maybe even for the first time.

**Q: Is there a time when it would be appropriate for the therapist to encourage the loved one to stay in the relationship?**

A: One of our primary tasks as the therapist is to model integral and congruent behavior. This means that we will be honest and up front as possible with a client if they may be pursuing a path – from a clinical perspective – that is not in their best interest. This does not mean that we should overly influence or manipulate their decision(s), rather lay out considerations and rationale behind encouraging them to stay in the relationship and continue to heal when possible. An example of this might be an absence of overt or covert abuse or safety issues present in the relationship and the addict is being honest and diligent in their recovery work. In this case, it might benefit the client to give the healing process some time and see if things get better. Ultimately, however, the choice to leave should be honored if that is what the partner chooses to do.

**Q: I like to send clients to Al-Anon or CoDA 12-step support groups. Is that still recommended?**

A: The authors are very encouraging of all clients seeking out and attending any useful support groups – including Al-Anon and ACA where useful. Supportive environments where people come together with peers (a cohort) is one of the most effective and engaging places to learn, make friendships, and find peace by spending time with "people just like me." *However, the authors do not refer individuals to such 12-step or related programs until they clearly understand that they are not responsible for another's addiction, nor can they ever contribute to an addict's choice to use or act out.* Support, hope, direction, guidance, and compassion are meant to be the focus of such groups, not blame or shame or "looking for what you did wrong." Clients who attend Al-Anon should be able to take what they like and leave the rest before they are ready to attend. They need guidance toward what messages and direction will help them grow as opposed to leave them doubting themselves. The focus in such environments should always rest upon the loved one's "obsession with the disease of addiction," in whatever form it takes. But their focus should never be about some kind of "addiction to the one they love." We do not recommend any referrals to CoDA for obvious reasons.

**Q: What about those who are so needy and desperate in close relationships that they become unable to function without one? Aren't they deeply Codependent?**

A: For several decades, the Diagnostic and Statistical Manual of Mental Disorders (the DSM) has had a fully fleshed out, criteria-based diagnosis for people who are so emotionally limited and impaired that they "cling" to other people for their own emotional stability. It's called dependent personality disorder. Sadly, DPD and Codependence are often conflated. Simply go online to look up the word "Codependency" and you will see the many ways and places where that same language has been conflated with terms like DPD, this, even though there are no formalized, universal measures that can be used to define Codependent people. Preexisting terms like DPD have clear, defined research-based diagnostic criteria created to help identify such pathologies.

**Q: What kind of treatment should be offered to loved ones of addicts? Don't they still need help with boundaries, self-care, and managing their situations?**

A: Loving persons in a meaningful relationship with an active addict are, by definition, in need of support. They likely need encouragement toward both greater self-care and establishing healthy boundaries with their troubled loved one. They need hope, direction, and insight into their problem. However, *no loving person in a meaningful relationship with an active addict should ever be asked to doubt the nature of their love, or to question their own emotional stability as a contributor to the addict's problems.*

**Q: What do you say to the millions of people who have embraced the concept of Codependence? Where does Prodependence leave these individuals?**

A  Taking the path of self-exploration and personal growth is a positive thing that strengthens individuals and society. We are certain that many of those who have embraced Codependence have become better people for having done so, and that is to be applauded. We would simply ask such individuals to reconsider the concept of "loving too much," as we see that the phrase as demeaning. For example, you may love in the wrong ways for the wrong reasons. You may love in ways that don't achieve the result you seek. You may love and lose. You may love and hurt. However, you can never feel too much love, express too much compassion, or exhibit too much empathy and if you do – the authors would like to claim you as a friend. To state that one can "love too much" remain in a relationship to an addicted person *as a reflection of their own pathology* is counterintuitive to our understanding into healthy human attachment and bonding. Endless research also tells us that by deepening and exploring our family and spousal intimacy, humans are much more likely to achieve self-actualization and personal growth than would be possible alone.

# Prodependence Clinical Guide List of References

Ainsworth, M. D. S., & Bowlby, J. (1991). An ethological approach to personality development. *American Psychologist, 46*(4), 333.

Alexander, B. K., Beyerstein, B. L., Hadaway, P. F., & Coambs, R. B. (1981). Effect of early and later colony housing on oral ingestion of morphine in rats. *Pharmacology Biochemistry and Behavior, 15*(4), 571–576.

American Psychiatric Association. (2013). *Diagnostic and statistical manual of mental disorders* (DSM-5®). American Psychiatric Publishing.

Barlow, M. R., Goldsmith Turrow, R. E., & Gerhart, J. (2017). Trauma appraisals, emotion regulation difficulties, and self-compassion predict posttraumatic stress symptoms following childhood abuse. *Child Abuse and Neglect, 65*, 37–47.

Barrell, A. (2020). Five breathing exercises for anxiety and how to do them. *Medical News Today*. www.medicalnewstoday.com/articles/breathing-exercises-for-anxiety

Beattie, M. (1986). *Codependent no more: How to stop controlling others and start caring for yourself*. Hazelden.

Bejerot, N. (1980). Addiction to pleasure: A biological and social-psychological theory of addiction. *NIDA Research Monograph, 30*, 246.

Black, C. (1981). *It will never happen to me: Children of alcoholics as youngsters–adolescents–adults*. Ballantine Books.

Blehar, M. C., Lieberman, A. F., & Ainsworth, M. D. S. (1977). Early face-to-face interaction and its relation to later infant-mother attachment. *Child Development, 48*(1), 182–194.

Books, B., & Bowlby, J. (1973). *Separation: Anxiety and anger* (Attachment and loss: Vol. 2). Hogarth Press.

Bowlby, J. (1988). *A secure base: Parent-child attachment and healthy human development*. Basic Books.

Brown, B. (2010). *The gifts of imperfection*. Hazelden Publishing.

Brown, B. (2012). *Daring greatly*. Penguin Random House.

Caspi, A., Harrington, H., Moffitt, T. E., Milne, B. J., & Poulton, R. (2006). Socially isolated children 20 years later: Risk of cardiovascular disease. *Archives of Pediatrics & Adolescent Medicine, 160*(8), 805–811.

Cermak, T. L. (1986). *Diagnosing and treating co-dependence: A guide for professionals who work with chemical dependents, their spouses and children*. Johnson Institute Books.

Coan, J. A., Schaefer, H. S., & Davidson, R. J. (2006). Lending a hand social regulation of the neural response to threat. *Psychological Science, 17*(12), 1032–1039.

Cohen, S. (2001). Social relationships and susceptibility to the common cold. *Emotion, Social Relationships, and Health*, 221–223.

Cohen, S., Doyle, W. J., Skoner, D. P., Rabin, B. S., & Gwaltney, J. M. (1997). Social ties and susceptibility to the common cold. *JAMA, 277*(24), 1940–1944.

Cowan, G., & Warren, L. W. (1994). Codependency and gender-stereotyped traits. *Sex Roles, 30*(9), 631–645.

Coyne, J. C., Rohrbaugh, M. J., Shoham, V., Sonnega, J. S., Nicklas, J. M., & Cranford, J. A. (2001). Prognostic importance of marital quality for survival of congestive heart failure. *The American Journal of Cardiology, 88*(5), 526–529.

Darwin, C. (1909). *The origin of species*. Dent.

Dear, G. E., & Roberts, C. M. (2002). The relationships between codependency and femininity and masculinity. *Sex Roles, 46*(5), 159–165.

Dorahy, M. J., Corry, M., Shannon, M., Webb, K., McDermott, B., Ryan, M., & Dyer, E. F. W. (2013). Complex trauma and intimate relationships: The impact of shame, guilt and dissociation. *Journal of Affective Disorders, 147*, 72–79.

Elliott, D. E., Bjelajac, P., Fallot, R. D., Markoff, L. S., & Reed, B. G. (2005). Trauma-informed or trauma-denied: Principles and implementation of trauma-informed services for women. *Journal of Community Psychology, 33*(4), 461–477.

Feeney, B. C. (2007). The dependency paradox in close relationships: Accepting dependence promotes independence. *Journal of Personality and Social Psychology, 92*(2), 268.

Frankl, V. E. L. (1992). *Man's search for meaning: An introduction to logotherapy* (4th ed.). Beacon Press.

Geller, J. D., & Farber, B. A. (2015). Attachment style, representations of psychotherapy, and clinical interventions with insecurely attached clients. *Journal of Clinical Psychology, 71*(5), 457–468.

Haaken, J. (1990). A critical analysis of the co-dependence construct. *Psychiatry, 53*(4), 396–406.

Hawkley, L. C., Masi, C. M., Berry, J. D., & Cacioppo, J. T. (2006). Loneliness is a unique predictor of age-related differences in systolic blood pressure. *Psychology and Aging, 21*(1), 152.

Hawkley, L. C., Thisted, R. A., Masi, C. M., & Cacioppo, J. T. (2010). Loneliness predicts increased blood pressure: 5-year cross-lagged analyses in middle-aged and older adults. *Psychology and Aging, 25*(1), 132.

Holmes, J. (2014). *John Bowlby and attachment theory (makers of modern psychotherapy)* (2nd ed.) [E-book]. Routledge.

Holt-Lunstad, J., Smith, T. B., & Layton, J. B. (2010). Social relationships and mortality risk: A meta-analytic review. *PLoS Medicine, 7*(7), e1000316.

House, J. S. (2001). Social isolation kills, but how and why? *Psychosomatic Medicine, 63*(2), 273–274.

House, J. S., Landis, K. R., & Umberson, D. (1988). Social relationships and health. *Science, 241*(4865), 540.

James, R., & Gilliland, B. (2012). *Crisis intervention strategies*. Nelson Education.

Johnson, S. M. (2004). *The practice of emotionally focused couples therapy* (2nd ed.). Taylor & Francis.

Johnson, S. M. (2008). *Hold me tight: Seven conversations for a lifetime of love*. Little, Brown.

Johnson, S. M. (2019). *Attachment theory in practice*. The Guilford Press.

Kavan, M., Guck, T., & Barone, E. (2006). A practical guide to crisis management. *American Family Physician, 74*(7), 1159–1164.

Kiecolt-Glaser, J. K., Malarkey, W. B., Chee, M., Newton, T., Cacioppo, J. T., Mao, H. Y., & Glaser, R. (1993). Negative behavior during marital conflict is associated with immunological down-regulation. *Psychosomatic Medicine, 55*(5), 395–409.

Kiecolt-Glaser, J. K., Newton, T., Cacioppo, J. T., MacCallum, R. C., Glaser, R., & Malarkey, W. B. (1996). Marital conflict and endocrine function: Are men really more physiologically affected than women? *Journal of Consulting and Clinical Psychology, 64*(2), 324.

Kübler-Ross, E., & Kessler, D. (2005). *On grief and grieving: Finding the meaning of grief through the five stages of loss.* Simon & Schuster.

Levine, A., & Heller, R. (2019). *Attached: Are you anxious, avoidant or secure? How the science of adult attachment can help you find – and keep – love* (Main Market ed.). Bluebird.

Luo, Y., Hawkley, L. C., Waite, L. J., & Cacioppo, J. T. (2012). Loneliness, health, and mortality in old age: A national longitudinal study. *Social Science & Medicine, 74*(6), 907–914.

Makinen, J. A., & Johnson, S. M. (2006). Resolving attachment injuries in couples using emotionally focused therapy: Steps toward forgiveness and reconciliation: Attachment theory and psychotherapy. *Journal of Consulting and Clinical Psychology, 74*(6), 1055–1064.

Mellody, P., Miller, A. W., & Miller, J. K. (1989). *Facing Codependence: What it is, where it comes from, how it sabotages our lives.* Harper Collins.

Merrill, S. M. (2018). *An exploration of the transition from romantic infatuation to adult attachment.* ProQuest Dissertations Publishing.

Neff, K. (2011). *Self-compassion: The proven power of being kind to yourself.* William Morrow.

Norwood, R. (1986). *Women who love too much: When you keep wishing and hoping he'll change.* Simon & Schuster.

Patterson, A. C., & Veenstra, G. (2010). Loneliness and risk of mortality: A longitudinal investigation in Alameda County, California. *Social Science & Medicine, 71*(1), 181–186.

Pekovic, V., Seff, L., & Rothman, M. (2007). Planning for and responding to special needs of elders in natural disasters. *Generations, 31*(4), 37–41.

Perissinotto, C. M., Cenzer, I. S., & Covinsky, K. E. (2012). Loneliness in older persons: A predictor of functional decline and death. *Archives of Internal Medicine, 172*(14), 1078–1084.

Platt, M. G., Luoma, J. B., & Freyd, J. J. (2016). Shame and dissociation in survivors of high and low betrayal trauma. *Journal of Aggression, Maltreatment & Trauma, 26*(1), 34–49.

Roberts, A. R. (2002). Assessment, crisis intervention, and trauma treatment: The integrative ACT intervention model. *Brief Treatment and Crisis Intervention, 2*(1), 1–22.

Rosenberg, R. A. (2013). *The history of the term codependency.* https://blogs.psychcentral.com/human-magnets/2013/11/the-history-of-the-term-codependency/

Rosenberg, R. A. (2018). *The human magnet syndrome: The codependent narcissist trap.* CreateSpace Independent Publishing.

Schaef, A.W. (1986). *Codependence: Misunderstood-mistreated.* HarperCollins.

Semenza, J. C., Rubin, C. H., Falter, K. H., Selanikio, J. D., Flanders, W. D., Howe, H. L., & Wilhelm, J. L. (1996). Heat-related deaths during the July 1995 heat wave in Chicago. *New England Journal of Medicine, 335*(2), 84–90.

Shepard, M. F., & Campbell, J. A. (1992). The Abusive Behavior Inventory: A measure of psychological and physical abuse. *Journal of Interpersonal Violence, 7*(3), 291–305. https://doi.org/10.1177/088626092007003001

Solomon, M., & Gullickson, T. (1995). *Lean on me: The power of positive dependency in intimate relationships.* Simon and Schuster: New York, 1994, p. 44.

Tatkin, S. (2012). *Wired for love: How understanding your partner's brain and attachment style can help you defuse conflict and build a secure relationship.* New Harbinger Publications.

Tatkin, S. (2018). *We do: Saying yes to a relationship of depth, true connection, and enduring love.* Sounds True.

The Therapist. (2020). Understanding mental health stigma in Black and Hispanic/Hispanic communities: An interview with Marianne Diaz and Eric Katende. *The Therapist, 2020,* 16–19.

Thomas, A. (1989) Drawing the line at safety. *History Today, 39*(2), 5–7.

Thurston, R. C., & Kubzansky, L. D. (2009). Women, loneliness, and incident coronary heart disease. *Psychosomatic Medicine, 71*(8), 836.

U.S. Department of Health and Human Services. (2009). *Results from the 2007 National Survey on Drug Use and Health: Detailed tables.* Substance Abuse and Mental Health Services Administration. SAMHSA, Office of Applied Studies.

Vaillant, G. E. (2008). *Aging well: Surprising guideposts to a happier life from the landmark study of adult development.* Hachette UK.

Weiss, R. (2018). *Prodependence: Moving beyond Codependency.* Health Communications, Inc.

Weiss, R. (2019). Prodependence vs. codependency: Would a new model (Prodependence) for treating loved ones of sex addicts be more effective than the model we've got (codependency)? *Sexual Addiction & Compulsivity, 26*(3–4), 177–190.

White, W., & Savage, B. (2005). All in the family: Alcohol and other drug problems, recovery advocacy. *Alcoholism Treatment Quarterly, 23*(4), 3–37.

Wikipedia. *Dependent personality disorder.* Retrieved March 8, 2018, from https://en.wikipedia.org/wiki/Dependent_personality_disorder

Woititz, J. G. (1990). *Adult children of alcoholics: Expanded edition.* Health Communications, Inc.

Wolfe, T. (1976). The me decade and the third great awakening. *New York Magazine, 23*(8), 26–40.

# Index

Printed in the United States
by Baker & Taylor Publisher Services